SOD IT!
EAT WELL

HEALTHY EATING INTO YOUR SIXTIES, SEVENTIES AND BEYOND

CONTENTS

INTRODUCTION

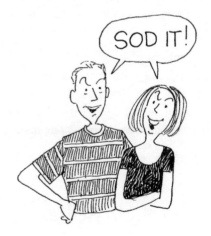

Well, you've made it into your sixties, seventies or eighties, so you obviously know a bit about what to eat already – but this book will help you eat even better and stay healthier for longer. In fact, if you follow our advice you will feel younger, like you did five or ten years ago. This is not because we are providing the recipe for the elixir of life; there is no magic substance or food that will reverse, stop or even slow down the ageing process. Of course, that doesn't stop people trying to find one; the main headline of the *Daily Express* recently was: 'Pill that adds 10 years to your life could be ready in a decade'... but don't hold your breath. But the good news is that there are other ways of dealing with the changes that too many of us still assume to be the inevitable consequences of ageing. The ageing process is natural and is not actually the cause of most of the problems that are attributed to it; if you were only affected by the ageing process you would be independent and active at the age of ninety. In reality, there are three other processes that affect us as we grow older:

- loss of fitness
- disease – caused not by the ageing process but by our environment and lifestyle, including what we eat
- adopting a negative attitude – based on the undue pessimism about old age that pervades our society

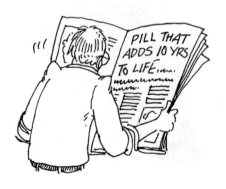

We now know that our lifespan – or length of life – and even more importantly our 'health span' – years of life free from disability – are much more determined by these three processes than by the ageing process.

Obviously it is best to maintain fitness, reduce the risk of disease and be positive throughout our lives. But it is particularly important when the phase of growth and development stops and the ageing process begins, which is about the age of thirty. However, the best news is that it is never too late to start and to enjoy the benefits that result from our efforts. Whether you are sixty or seventy or eighty, you can do yourself the world of good if you follow these simple steps:

- keep active physically to improve and maintain your bodily fitness
- keep active mentally
- stay involved and use your experience to help others
- stop smoking – try again even if you have failed ten times
- use medicines and healthcare with caution, and only if you develop disease
- eat well – the subject of this book

If you want to learn about the first five steps listed here then read *Sod Sixty!* and *Sod Seventy!*, the companion books to this one. The word 'sod' was chosen for the titles of these books because it expressed the anger and irritation of the author on being asked by a younger person in rather gloating fashion and for the umpteenth time: 'How does it feel to be sixty?' He replied: 'Sod sixty, sod that, you just have to get a ****** grip.'

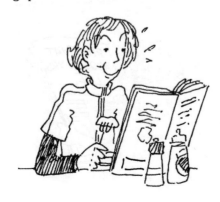

The people who asked the question were scientifically trained, some of them as medical doctors. The author's exasperation was due to the fact that he thought everyone knew that being sixty or seventy is not a matter of how you feel. Of course feelings are important, but how you are at sixty or seventy really depends on what you have done to keep healthy in the previous decade, what your outlook is on the next and a little bit of good luck. Your genes are important but determine only about 20 per cent of your health. In any case your genes and your environment are interwoven. You need to be lucky enough to have inherited fewer than average of the genes that cause, or increase the risk of disease. You also need to be lucky enough to be born into a family that is stable, wealthy, not stinking rich but not impoverished, and which values children and their education. We now know that the environment in which your parents and even your grandparents lived can influence the way your genes work. However, once again this only determines another 20 per cent of the state of your health. The other factors, which are under your control (and they're worth repeating), are:

- your physical activity
- your mental activity
- how engaged you are in helping other people
- your lifestyle, for example whether you smoke, or drink too much alcohol
- how you cope with disease and use healthcare wisely
- what you eat

The 'sod sixty' comment was the result of what has been called the Curse of Knowledge, which in essence is the problem that someone who has been learning about a particular thing for years has trouble remembering what it was like not to know about that thing. Stupidly, the exasperated sixty-year-old had overlooked the fact that it had taken him more than ten years to learn and accept that ageing was relatively unimportant and that the three other factors had to be taken into account.

The comment was not an insult addressed to the individual who had asked the question 'how does it feel to be sixty?' once too often, even though it was a little annoying, it was actually directed at the idea that being sixty means being old. In retrospect the comment seemed so appropriate that 'sod it' has become the general term we use to put ideas that some people associate with being sixty, seventy or older, in their place. These include ideas such as:

- old people are conservative and don't like change
- people aged sixty should just take it easy
- people aged sixty or seventy have had it good and we are now paying for their pensions
- fitness is only for young people
- all older people are demented
- all old people are the same
- everything that happens to older people is due to the ageing process

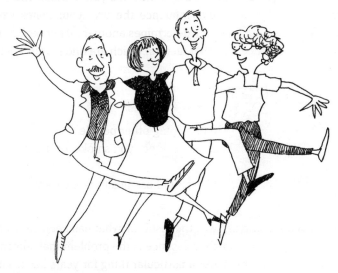

Sadly, these and other great 'myths of ageing', described in a book of that title by Joan T. Erber, are not only held by people who have been poorly educated, they are the beliefs held by many educated people, including some health care professionals and even doctors. It was for this reason that *Sod Sixty!* and *Sod Seventy!* were conceived and written. The core message in both books is the same, but there are important differences. For example, those in their sixties were born in the 1950s, those in their seventies in the 1940s; those in their sixties are often still caring for parents in their nineties; those in their seventies may be caring for a spouse or friend who has become disabled by disease.

Many of the issues faced by those born in the baby-boom era are dealt with in the two earlier titles but the topic of eating well in your sixties and beyond needed its own edition; hence the book you are holding in your hands. The problem is not ignorance. Many people are not aware that the risk of dementia can be reduced by about 30 per cent by doing exactly what we are advocating here, but when they are informed they pick it up quickly. In matters to do with food, eating and diet there is a different problem – confusion.

Every year a new 'guru' appears with a revolutionary 'diet' that will transform your life, an expert in the medical or healthcare establishment issues new guidelines on this or that food type and, understandably, every doctor and nurse seems to have their own position on eggs or cholesterol or statins. There is agreement on some things, on Five A Day for example, but in comparison with professional knowledge and advice on smoking – Stop It – or exercise – Increase It – knowledge about, and advice on, diet is at best confused and at worst contradictory. If you add the confusion about ageing you get in a right mess – and that is why we have written this book. The professionals are equally confused except for the excellent registered nutritionists and dietitians, but there are far too few of them to go round. In October 2015, NICE, the key source of evidence and guidance for the NHS and public health in England, published a major report emphasising that 'disability, dementia and frailty' were all preventable by actions taken in midlife, the main one being a healthy diet that included eating fruit and vegetables daily. The result in their view is 'healthy ageing'.

What we have tried to do is to draw on the scientific evidence about nutrition and diet and to imagine how we can help you think about the options you face, and the obstacles you have to overcome to eat well. Where can you turn for advice? Well, we recommend NHS Choices – www.nhs.uk - and this book!

It is aimed at people who are sixty or older and our aim is to explain how what you eat can counter many of the problems that people assume are caused by 'old age' and how changing your diet can help you:

- feel younger
- look younger if you are overweight

- reduce the risk of disease and disability
- stay healthier longer
- live longer
- enjoy food even more

We would like to start by asking you to reflect on your diet and on your relationship with food and eating. Let's start with some practical information about what you, or your nearest and dearest, actually eat.

What I eat, honestly

No one is checking this, so be honest with yourself. In the table below indicate how often in a typical week at home – not on holiday or at Christmas – you eat the following foods:

	Never	Some days	Most days	Every day
Crisps and snacks				
Chocolates or sweets				
Cakes and biscuits				
Puddings				
Sweetened drinks, e.g. squash, fizzy drinks, juice, sweetened coffee or tea				
Pizza, ready meals				
Takeaways				

If you ticked 'most days' or 'every day' to more than one of the categories, then you're probably getting too much sugar and salt, insufficient fibre and your diet is likely to be out of balance. You really would benefit from making some changes to your eating habits. The good news is that you don't have to drastically overhaul your diet or embark on a gruelling exercise regime to reap the benefits of a healthy diet. Just making some small changes can help you feel better and enjoy better health.

Your relationship with food

What you get from this book will depend not only on the information it contains but also on the attitudes, interests and habits that you bring to the subject of food and eating. In order to find out a little about this here are a few more questions that you should be asking yourself before you start reading in earnest.

We could start by asking if you are male or female, but you know the answer to that. Despite the fact that many of our celebrity chefs are men, it is fair to say that the average British male is not known for his cooking skills. This needs to change and we hope this book will help the man who is reading it, the woman who is choosing to buy a copy as a present for a man they love as well as those women looking for a good place to find some fresh culinary inspiration.

Central to all this is your relationship with food and eating – please note that this is your 'relationship' with food *and* eating. The two are independent, but obviously closely related. The first thing you must do is find out where you stand on the spectrum below:

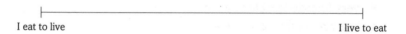

I eat to live   I live to eat

Some people are not particularly interested in food, never watch cookery programmes on TV and eat what they like, hopefully in moderation. Others are very interested in food, watch all the programmes, cook new recipes regularly and save up to go out and eat in restaurants, not only to avoid the bother of cooking and washing up but also for the experience of trying new tastes. We presume you belong to the latter group or you would not have bought this book.

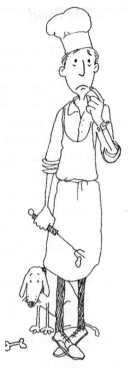

But let's delve a little deeper. Would you say you were:

- very knowledgeable about diet and health?
- knew more than average about how to eat for better health?
- confused by the dietary advice you get from the media?

Would you like to:

- learn more about food and how it can help you to better health?
- learn new recipes?
- lose weight?
- help someone else lose weight?

There's one more thing. Think for a moment about your own situation. Life changes as we get older and it is essential that we adapt our eating habits accordingly. If any of the following changes have occurred in your life recently then it's high time you took them into account:

- have you changed your lifestyle recently, for example, by retiring?

- if you are still working does your job involve:

    standing all the time?
    sitting all the time?
    maybe a bit of both?

- do you live on your own? It is much harder to motivate yourself to learn new recipes if it is only you eating them, but you can start inviting people over to share your cooking

- do you grow any of your own vegetables or herbs? If not, why not?

Answering these questions will help you decide what you want from this book. The fact is, eating well is vitally important at any age and never more so than in your sixties and beyond. What you eat now can make a big difference to how you feel, how much energy you have, your ability to ward off illnesses – and even to your appearance. In short, eating well will vastly increase your chances of living a longer and healthier life! And it's never too late to start.

This book will show you how to make simple changes to your diet and reap the rewards in terms of better health. It's written in a Q&A style – this means the vast subject of nutrition is broken down into more manageable chunks, making the whole thing (excuse the pun) easier to swallow. And, in addition to all the vital nutritional information, you'll find lots about the latest nutritional research. In other words, it's topical as well as practical. We hope that by the time you finish reading this book you will have all the information and confidence you need to make sure you're eating the right combination of foods to keep you fit, happy and well.

And one final thing. Less men cook in the home than women, do the weekly shop, or plan meals – but often have more nutritional problems than women. The solution? It's time for those men who still don't to do their fair share - planning, preparing and cooking at least one meal a day. There may be some unrecognised Gordon Ramsay or Heston Blumenthal out there, but even if there is not, men must start to take a deeper interest in food – it is one of the means by which they can live a longer and, of even greater importance, healthier life.

Muir Gray and Anita Bean

WHAT TO EAT

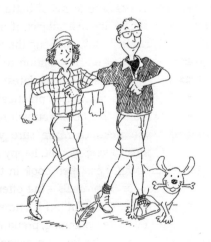

We've never had so much information about food, diet and health available to us. Newspapers are full of the latest diet fixes and fads, the internet is awash with miracle food cures and there's no end of so-called experts telling us 'Don't eat this, don't eat that!' The trouble is much of the information available seems contradictory and confusing, so knowing what to eat and what to avoid can be a bit of a minefield. One day we're told red wine and chocolate are good for us and the next we learn that they're bad. Low fat foods that we once thought were healthy turn out to be loaded with sugar and worse for us than the original high fat versions. It's the same with fruit juices and smoothies — once regarded as good for us, experts now say they can be as bad for our teeth and waistlines as cola. And, although food labels are a good idea, they are often so confusing we are still in the dark as to just how good or bad certain foods are for us. On top of that, we're constantly bombarded by food adverts, special offers and promotions, making it impossible to resist temptation in the supermarket.

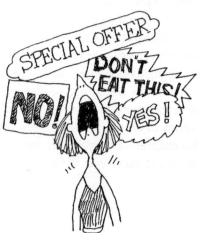

Maybe you're confused about how much fat and carbohydrate you need to eat and whether saturated fats really are bad for your heart after all. Is butter better for you than margarine? Then what about the salt content of our food? Why is salt so harmful and how can we cut down our intake?

The danger of all this conflicting information is that we take it with – forgive me, another pun – a pinch of salt and then ignore really sound advice. Yes, it's difficult to see the wood for the trees sometimes. But have no fear. This book is here to help – to remind you of the main rules, to debunk the myths and help you sort the facts from the fiction.

Let's get one thing straight – food is one of the great joys of life and should never be treated as the enemy. You don't need to go on a diet or give up your favourite foods. Diets don't work and banning any food inevitably leads to craving and over-indulgence. What you need to do is strike the right balance in what you're eating. It's all about common sense and making small changes, rather than attempting a completely new way of eating. That way you're more likely to stick to your new healthy habits and, before you know it, eating well will become a way of life.

This chapter is all about giving you the information and the knowledge you need to have the healthiest possible eating plan; one that will last you for the rest of your life. It will show you how to make a few simple tweaks to your diet that can help you improve your health. Ultimately, a healthy diet means eating a wide variety of nutrient-packed foods, focusing on unprocessed and fresh foods wherever possible, avoiding too much sugar, fat and salt and keeping highly processed foods to a minimum – very much along the lines of the traditional Mediterranean diet (which we describe and recommend in Chapter 2). Don't worry about getting bogged down in all the science and research behind the information in this chapter – the important thing is that we're here to arm you with all the facts you need to make the right food choices for life.

Calories

As we get older, our nutritional needs and dietary requirements change. This is due mainly to the fact that we are less active than we once were and so burn fewer calories. And that means you have to adjust your food intake in order to avoid putting on weight.

How many calories should you eat?

How much you should eat depends on how active you are. If you eat more calories than your body uses, you gain weight. You don't need to get bogged down counting calories but knowing roughly how many you need may help you make better sense of the calories you see on food labels, and help you keep a check on portion sizes. As a rough guide:

A woman over 60 who is ...

- not physically active needs about 1600 calories a day
- somewhat physically active needs about 1800 calories a day
- very active needs about 2000 calories a day

A man over 60 who is ...

- not physically active needs about 2000 calories a day
- somewhat physically active needs about 2200–2400 calories a day
- very active needs about 2400–2800 calories a day

Source: *National Institute of Aging*

Why do you need fewer calories as you get older?

As we get older lots of us become less active, which causes a loss of muscle tissue and a corresponding drop in the number of calories you burn at rest and during activity. But this isn't inevitable. Regular exercise (especially resistance training exercises, such as push-ups, resistance band or dumb-bell exercises) can help reduce or even prevent this. And this is a key feature of the 5S fitness programme outlined in *Sod Seventy!*. Doing just ten minutes a day of strength-focused exercise along with three longer sessions a week of stamina-focused exercises (like walking or cycling) will not only maintain your fitness in your 60s, 70s and beyond, but will also prevent muscle loss. The key is to get – and keep – moving!

Why do men need more calories than women?

Men generally have higher calorie requirements than women because they have more muscle tissue and, generally, weigh more. Muscle tissue has a big appetite for calories. The more muscle mass you have, the more calories you will burn. And the heavier you are (whether that's muscle or fat), the higher your metabolic rate (the number of calories you burn, see page 100).

Fat

Fat was once regarded as 'the enemy' – something to avoid at all costs – but *that's no longer the case*. On the contrary, your body needs fat as it plays a critical role in heart health as well as providing fuel and helping to keep cell membranes healthy. Fat in food also provides essential omega-3 and omega-6 polyunsaturated fatty acids, which help keep your heart healthy, and the fat-soluble vitamins A, D and E, which are good for your skin, bones and overall well-being. What's more, fat in foods gives the body the feeling of being full and therefore satisfies your appetite. A diet that contains very little fat can leave you feeling hungry.

All fats are high in calories (compared with carbohydrate and protein) and it's important to bear this in mind if you are watching your weight. However, this doesn't mean you have to cut it out from your diet completely. Gone are the days of extremely low fat diets. Studies have shown that diets containing moderate amounts of fat (such as the Mediterranean diet, universally recommended by nutrition experts for a longer, healthier and happier life) are more effective than low fat diets in protecting against heart disease, stroke, type 2 diabetes, high blood cholesterol and high blood pressure. They have also been shown to help with healthy weight loss.

How much fat should you eat?

The National Health Service (NHS) recommends that fat makes up 20–35 per cent of your daily energy (calorie) intake. This means the average man on a 2000-calorie diet should eat approximately 44g–78g of fat a day, equivalent to about 4 tablespoons of olive oil (we'll show you how you can hit your fat target on page 16). But it's just as important to pay attention to the type of fat in your diet, as it is to monitor your total fat intake.

What are the different types of fat?

There are three main types of fat – saturated, monounsaturated and polyunsaturated – and most foods contain a combination of all three. Eat all fats in moderation, whether saturated or unsaturated.

Saturated fats

Saturated fats are mostly found in animal products (meat, sausages, burgers, bacon, egg yolk, butter, milk and cheese) as well as palm oil ('vegetable fat') and coconut oil. At the moment UK guidelines encourage us to swap some saturated for unsaturated fats. This is because diets high in saturated fat can raise levels of cholesterol. A high level of cholesterol is linked to an increased risk of heart disease. However, a major study of more than 600,000 people conducted in 2014, found no association between saturated fat and the risk of heart disease, which suggests that saturated fat may not be as harmful for your heart as once thought.

The jury is still out as to how much is safe but for now try to consume no more than 10 per cent energy (calories) from saturated fat, that's 20g a day on a 2000 calorie diet. Swapping some of the saturated fats in your diet for unsaturated fats can help lower cholesterol levels.

HOW MUCH SATURATED FAT SHOULD YOU EAT?

While saturated fat may not be as bad as once thought, it doesn't mean you can eat as much as you want. You still need to keep a check on calories and portion sizes.

Meat: stick to one or two servings (100–200g) a week, say Harvard University researchers, but avoid processed meats (such as bacon, sausages and ham) altogether if possible, as eating just 50g a day was associated with a 42 per cent increased risk of heart disease.

Whole milk: studies show that people who consume whole milk do better at keeping the pounds off than those drinking skimmed milk – possibly due to the higher levels of fat in whole milk that make us feel fuller for longer so we end up drinking less – but portions still matter, so drink no more than 3 cups per day.

Butter: it may be back in favour as a natural, minimally processed source of fat but it's still high in calories (745cal/100g), so keep portion sizes small (thinly spread on a slice of toast, for example).

Cheese: protein curbs hunger and keeps you feeling satisfied after meals, so cheese may help you eat less at your next meal, according to a study in the *British Journal of Nutrition*. Lowest calorie options are mozzarella, feta and goat's cheese.

Monounsaturated fats

These are the good guys – monounsaturated fats are found in olive oil, olives, avocados, nuts, seeds and rapeseed oil. They lower harmful LDL cholesterol levels without affecting 'good' HDL and can cut the risk of heart disease and cancer.

Eating a diet that is moderate in total fat but rich in monounsaturated fats (such as the traditional Mediterranean diet) is thought to be healthier than a low fat diet, reducing the risk of heart disease and stroke. A study published in 2013 found that those eating a Mediterranean-style diet that included large amounts of olive oil or nuts cut their risk of suffering a heart attack or stroke by 30 per cent compared with those following a conventional low fat diet.

Polyunsaturated fats

Found in sunflower oil, corn oil, safflower oil (emerging as a new choice of healthy cooking oil and available at many supermarkets), sunflower oil margarine, nuts and seeds, polyunsaturated fats are also good for you. Two types in particular – the omega-3 and omega-6 fatty acids – are called 'essential fatty acids' because they are needed in your diet to help maintain the correct structure of cell membranes in the body. The one problem is that our bodies cannot produce them.

Omega-3 fats

These unsaturated fats, found primarily in oily fish, have a wide range of benefits, including regulating blood pressure, blood clotting and boosting immunity, as well as possibly reducing the risk of heart disease and stroke, symptoms in rheumatoid arthritis and slowing the progression of age-related macular degeneration (AMD), a disease of reduced vision. According to recent research, omega-3s may also help prevent Alzheimer's disease and treat depression.

You only need small amounts of omega-3 fatty acids to keep you healthy. The NHS recommends one portion (140g) of oily fish, such as sardines, mackerel, salmon, fresh (not tinned) tuna, trout and herring, per week (see www.nhs.uk). If you don't like oily fish, you can get omega-3 fats from walnuts, pumpkin seeds, flaxseed oil, rapeseed oil and omega-3 eggs (which come from hens fed on an omega-3 enriched diet).

Omega-3 supplements are widely available, but it is preferable to get yours from food sources. There is little evidence that supplements protect you from heart disease or other chronic diseases. What's more, omega-3 supplements may also be unsuitable for people with certain conditions and may interact with some medicines including those that control high blood pressure. If you are thinking of taking a fish oil supplement, it's best to speak to your doctor.

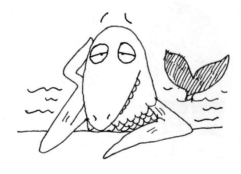

Omega-6 fats

Omega-6 fatty acids are found in a wide variety of foods, including vegetable oils such as soya, corn, safflower, sunflower and groundnut oil, margarine and foods made with these oils. For this reason, most people currently eat too much omega-6 in relation to omega-3, which can result in an imbalance of certain hormones and chronic inflammation. Inflammation has been linked to cardiovascular disease, arthritis, stroke and cancer.

Limit your intake of processed and deep-fried foods, and use oils that are rich in monounsaturated fats, such as olive oil and rapeseed oil instead of omega-6-rich vegetable and seed oils such as corn, safflower and sunflower oil.

Trans fats

These really are the bogeymen of the fat world – avoid them wherever possible. Trans fats are a type of unsaturated fat that behave like saturated fat because of their chemical structure. They are found in hydrogenated fat, formed when hydrogen is added to liquid oils to make them solid. They increase blood levels of LDL cholesterol ('bad' cholesterol), harden your arteries and increase your risk of heart disease. Pressure from public health campaigners means manufacturers have removed these fats from many foods, but high levels can still be found in fast foods and takeaways, pies, pastries and bakery items, margarines, cereal bars and low quality chocolate (see Should I Eat… chocolate on page 29). Check the label for 'hydrogenated' or 'partially hydrogenated fat' and if you find these words then put the product down.

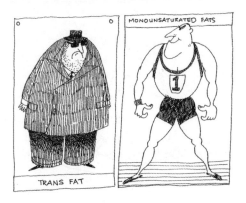

19

ARE LOW FAT DIETS GOOD FOR YOU?

No... low fat diets are a thing of the past. We now know that the world's healthiest populations eat a *moderate* fat diet that includes natural and healthy fats like olive oil, olives, nuts, fish and avocados. This style of eating, which in this book we've chosen to refer to as the traditional Mediterranean diet, is famously associated with lower rates of heart disease and stroke (see page 66). It is not a low fat diet but is still within the fat intake levels recommended by the NHS. The problem with low fat diets is that they're not very satisfying, so you're likely to get hungry and end up snacking on things like low fat cereal bars and biscuits – all of which are loaded with sugar and just as high in calories. This is a recipe for disaster if you're trying to shift the pounds. According to studies, low fat/high sugar diets can also push up blood fat levels, which raise – not lower – the risk of heart disease. Strike the right balance by including fish, olive oil and full-fat milk in your meals and snacking on nuts and seeds instead of biscuits.

SHOULD I EAT... BUTTER OR MARGARINE?

For a long time butter was a no-no (it was believed to increase your risk of heart disease) while margarine was thought to be the healthier option. But now the thinking has reversed and experts say butter is, in fact, *better for you*. For a start, it's an all-natural product (made from cream) whereas margarine is artificial, being made from cheap refined oils and additives. Secondly, the saturated fats in butter aren't quite as bad for the heart as once thought.

Spreads made with olive oil are perhaps a healthier option as they contain high levels of heart-healthy monounsaturated fats. As a bonus, they're also slightly lower in calories and fat than butter or margarine.

If you have high blood cholesterol levels, you may wish to opt for spreads containing plant stanols (e.g. Benecol and Flora Proactive). These can help stop cholesterol being absorbed from your food. Eating three servings a day may lower your cholesterol levels by between 7–10 per cent (one serving is 10g, the average amount spread on a slice of bread).

The cholesterol question

Cholesterol is a waxy substance, which forms part of the membrane that surrounds every cell in your body. It is also used to make hormones such as testosterone and oestrogen. Most of the cholesterol in the body is made in the liver and then sent to the cells that need it bound to a lipoprotein called LDL (low density lipoprotein). The amount of cholesterol you make depends on your genes, stress levels and the *amount of saturated fat you eat*. It is present in some foods such as eggs, offal and shellfish. However, for most people, the cholesterol in food has very little effect on blood cholesterol levels. What's important is the amount of saturated fat you eat. Once inside the body, the liver turns this fat into cholesterol. Having too much cholesterol in the blood pushes up your risk of heart disease and stroke.

Carbohydrate

Carbohydrate gives you energy for keeping your brain, nervous system and heart going as well as fuelling all your daily activities and exercise. Potatoes, pasta, rice, oats as well as beans, lentils and fruit are all 'carbs'. Exactly how much you need depends on how active you are – the more active you are, the more carbohydrate you will burn. For example, jogging, swimming or cycling burn more carbohydrate than walking, housework and gardening.

Of course, this isn't a licence to over-indulge in a big bowl of pasta every time you go out for a long walk or spend a bit of time cutting the lawn – in reality, even the very active probably won't need more than an extra potato or a couple of slices of bread to fill them up after exercise. Too much carbohydrate, of course, can lead to unwanted pounds (see Chapter 3). The NHS recommends we all get around half of our daily calories from carbohydrate.

It's best to get most of your daily carbohydrate quota from nutrient-packed, fibre-rich foods (or wholefoods) – wholegrains, potatoes, beans, lentils, fruit and vegetables – rather than sugary foods or highly processed foods stripped of fibre, such as white bread, pasta and rice, cakes, chocolates and biscuits. Wholefoods provide longer-lasting energy and help you feel full for longer. The easiest way to get the balance right is by eating mostly 'real' foods – simple meals made from scratch 'like your mother used to make' – rather than ready meals, takeaways and snacks.

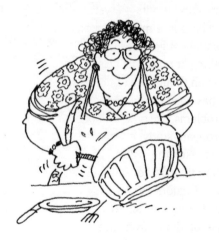

Sugar

Sugar is pure calories… unnecessary calories. It makes foods taste sweet but contains nothing nutritional, such as fibre, vitamins or minerals.

There are two main problems with sugar. Firstly, it increases the risk of tooth decay. Studies have shown that populations with the highest rate of tooth decay have the highest intakes of sugar; those with the lowest rates of decay consume very little sugar indeed. So cutting back on sugar will help to protect your teeth from decay.

CHILDREN AND SWEETS

Lots of grandparents like to spoil their grandchildren by giving them sweets and other sugary snacks. While there's nothing wrong with the odd treat – after all, that's what grandparents are for! – just make sure you don't overdo it. Sugar is especially harmful for children's teeth and too many sugary treats can store up problems of obesity and type 2 diabetes as they get older.

Secondly, sugar makes foods more tasty and easy to over-consume. In other words, it adds to the amount of calories in food without adding bulk. It is often found with lots of fat, for example, in chocolates, cakes, doughnuts and biscuits – a very 'moreish' combination. So it is all too easy to consume more calories than we realise and put on weight. Unfortunately, sugar doesn't fill us up or put the brakes on our appetite. If anything, it makes us want to eat and drink more – so we keep on eating even though we're not truly hungry. In studies, a high intake of sugar has been linked to obesity. And with obesity come all sorts of other problems, like type 2 diabetes, heart disease and cancer.

A 2015 European study concluded that drinking 1–2 sugary drinks a day increases the risk of type 2 diabetes by 26 per cent. A study published in 2014 revealed that those who consume more than 25 per cent of calories from added sugar* (that's equivalent to 31 teaspoons a day or four slices of cake for the average person) trebled their risk of dying from heart disease or stroke compared with those who consumed less than 10 per cent from added sugar (12 teaspoons a day). However, you don't need to ban sugar completely. If you're healthy, slim and active then *sugar in moderation* won't do you any harm – and you can still treat yourself to the occasional ice cream or slice of cake. But it's important to remember there's no need for 'added' sugars in the diet – they make food taste sweet but they don't serve any purpose apart from fuel (calories). The less you eat, the healthier you'll be.

* 'Added' sugars is a confusing term. In fact they are the sugars added to food and drink, as well as sugars that are naturally present in fruit

juice, syrups and honey. They're not the sugars found naturally in milk products, whole fruit and vegetables.

SHOULD I EAT... SUGAR OR HONEY?

Honey is mostly sugar (73 per cent) – plus water (27 per cent) – and counts towards your daily limit of added sugar (see page 25). However, it can be regarded as slightly less 'bad for you' than ordinary sugar. According to studies, it raises blood sugar* less than sugar does (due to its higher content of fructose) and also contains small amounts of antioxidants (darker honeys contain more than lighter varieties). So, if you like the taste, use it as an alternative to some of the sugar in your meals and in recipes. Its stronger flavour means you may be able to use a little less. Honey is used in many of the sweet recipes in Chapter 5 (see pages 201–208).

* 'Blood sugar' refers to the amount of glucose in your blood. Glucose is carried via the bloodstream to the body's cells where it is used for energy. Blood sugar concentration needs to be kept within a very narrow range: 70–110mg/100ml or 3.9–6.1mmol/l (millimoles per litre). This allows normal body functions to continue. If your blood sugar level drops below the normal range you will have 'low blood sugar' or hypoglycaemia (often called hypo) and you may experience dizziness, faintness or even pass out, because the brain isn't getting enough glucose.

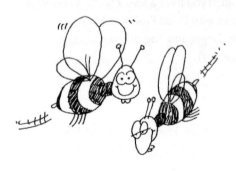

HOW MUCH SUGAR SHOULD YOU EAT?

Food experts recommend cutting down on the amount of sugar we eat. At the moment, we're eating on average 60g (15 teaspoons) daily, equivalent to two cupcakes or one and a half cans of fizzy drink, but the government recommends that we cut this by more than half, and aim to get no more than 25g (6 teaspoons on a 2000 calorie diet) from added sugar a day (or 5 per cent of calories). This is the amount in one cupcake or a small bar of chocolate. With these guidelines even drinking just one glass of orange juice and a slice of toast with jam would push you over the limit.

When buying food, check the label for words such as sucrose, glucose syrup, invert sugar and glucose. Even healthy sounding ingredients like maple syrup, agave nectar and honey are all forms of added sugar.

The easiest way to cut down on sugar is by eliminating sweetened drinks, like squash, cordial, juice drinks, fizzy drinks (such as cola or lemonade) and energy drinks.

Swap these sugary drinks for water, sugar-free drinks (such as no-added sugar squash or diet drinks) or unsweetened drinks (such as coffee and tea) whenever you can. If you put sugar in your coffee or tea, then cut down gradually, half a teaspoon at a time, to give your palate time to adjust.

Cutting sugar doesn't mean having to give up all your favourite sweet treats. Just eat less, and choose naturally sweet foods, like fruit, instead. If you have a sweet tooth and enjoy puddings try Baked Apples with Dried Fruit and Nuts (page 205), Poached Plums with Ginger and Yogurt (page 204) or Healthy Banana Bread (page 207).

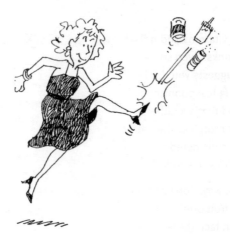

Are all sugars bad for you?

No they're not; the government target of 25g per day doesn't include sugars that occur naturally in foods such as milk (lactose), fruit and vegetables (fructose, glucose and sucrose), which are locked into the structure of the food. This makes them far less harmful to health than added sugar. That's because the sugars are much less concentrated and because the fibre present in the foods slows the absorption of the sugar into the body and so prevents a sharp rise in blood sugar and insulin. Also, these foods are very difficult to overeat. *You would need to eat three apples to get the same amount of sugar as in a big glass of apple juice.* The chances are you'd feel full before you could eat that many apples.

SHOULD I DRINK... FRUIT JUICE?

We used to think of fruit juice as a healthy option but, in fact, 'natural' sugars in fruit juices are no better for you than added sugars in soft drinks. Removing the fibre from an apple, for example, when you're making apple juice, means the sugars are more concentrated and absorbed very fast. It seems unbelievable, *but most juices contain as much sugar as cola.* For example, a standard glass (250ml) of apple juice contains 24g sugar while a glass of cola contains 26g. However, as fruit juices contain vitamins and minerals, they are healthier options than sugary drinks. Even so, be wary – the British Nutrition Foundation suggests you drink no more than one small glass (150ml) a day (3 teaspoons of sugar) to stay within the sugar guidelines. And that's a rather small glass by most people's standards! It's more like the amount we drank in the 70s when fruit juice was considered a 'luxury starter' in restaurants! Not the everyday drink it is today!

Oh, and by the way, don't be taken in by those fancy labels on 'sparkling' fruit drinks. They make the drink appear more 'natural' but, in fact, these drinks contain just as much sugar as fizzy drinks. For example, a single can of sparkling lemon drink can contain 33g – or 8 teaspoons – of sugar, more than the government's recommended daily limit.

Are artificial sweeteners better than sugar?

Despite bad press, aspartame, stevia, sucralose and other calorie-free sweeteners used in 'diet' or 'sugar free' drinks have all passed the scrutiny of food safety committees worldwide. And the latest research from the European Food Safety authority (EFSA) is that artificial sweeteners aren't linked with cancer. However, it is thought that they increase some people's desire for sweetness, so limiting them and having water instead of diet drinks is a good idea.

HOW MUCH SUGAR DO YOU EAT?

	Calories	Sugar (in grams)	Sugar (in teaspoons*)
2 scoops ice cream	215	16	4
1 can cola	139	35	9
1 glass cranberry juice drink	115	28	7
1 slice chocolate cake	355	21	5
1 glass apple juice	118	28	7

1 blueberry muffin (coffee shop)	448	28	7
1 small bar milk chocolate (32g)	263	27	7
1 cereal bar	170	9	2
2 chocolate biscuits	200	10	2½
1 jam doughnut	239	13	3
1 cup cake	143	15	4
1 small bowl crunchy nut cornflakes	121	11	3

*1 teaspoon = 4g sugar

How to cut sugar

Avoid these foods and drinks, in order of importance:

1. Soft drinks like cola, lemonade, sparkling juice drinks and energy drinks – these contain very high levels (around 35g (8 teaspoons) in an average can) and the sugar is rapidly absorbed.
2. Fruit juices – this may surprise you but they contain the same amount of sugar as soft drinks.
3. Sweets – provide sugar and nothing else.
4. Biscuits, cereal bars and cakes – these are high in sugar *and* fat.
5. Low-fat or reduced-fat foods – snacks, biscuits and desserts that have the fat removed are often very high in sugar to provide some pleasant taste.

 DO IT NOW!

Having read this section so far and come to the conclusion that you consume too much sugar, here are some useful suggestions to help you cut this over-consumption:

☑ drink water instead of soft drinks and fruit juice

☑ instead of having sugar in porridge, homemade drinks or stewed fruit, try cinnamon, nutmeg, vanilla, almond extract, ginger or lemon

☑ avoid processed foods and satisfy your sweet tooth with fresh fruit instead – try a fresh fruit salad or Summer Fruit Compote with Yogurt (page 208) or Roasted Peaches and Plums with Yogurt (page 202)

So, what can I have for breakfast if it's not cereal and fruit juice?

Shop-bought breakfast cereals can be extremely high in sugar. But there are some simple sugar swaps that'll help you cut down during that all-important first meal of the day. Instead of adding sugar to your cereal, try adding fruit such as strawberries and blueberries or dried fruit for a natural sweet fix. Alternatively, you could start your day with a warming bowl of porridge topped with fruit (see Berry Porridge, page 166, or Overnight Oats, page 170) or make your own sugar-free muesli (see Energy-Boosting Muesli, page 168, or Bircher Muesli, page 169). A good tip is whatever you choose to eat you can enhance foods with spices instead of sugar: try ginger, allspice, cinnamon or nutmeg in your porridge (see Cinnamon Porridge with Banana and Nuts, page 167). Another delicious meal could be plain Greek yogurt with chopped fresh fruit or dried fruit (see Blueberry and Almond Yogurt, page 171). Wash it all down with a glass of water and you'll be well set up for the day.

SHOULD I EAT... CHOCOLATE?

In some studies chocolate has been found to reduce blood pressure, improve mental performance and cut the risk of heart disease, stroke and certain cancers. But before you celebrate with a family-sized bar of milk chocolate, it's worth noting that the studies used chocolate (cocoa) *extracts*, not the commercial bars we buy in the shops, which, unfortunately, contain very little of the beneficial compounds (called polyphenols) found in cocoa extract. Dark chocolate with 70 per cent cocoa solids contains a little more than milk chocolate (along with iron and magnesium), but you would need to eat huge quantities to get a significant boost. Since dark and milk chocolate are both loaded with calories (about 500 calories per 100g), sugar (30g per 100g) and fat (14g per 100g), the weight gain risk outweighs the benefits. There are better options for getting your polyphenols, for example, tea, fruit, vegetables, red wine and nuts.

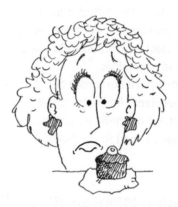

Fibre

Fibre helps promote healthy digestion by moving foods through the digestive tract. Foods rich in fibre, including wholegrains such as porridge and wholegrain pasta, beans, chickpeas, lentils, fruits, and vegetables, have other health benefits too, including preventing constipation, diverticular disease (when small pouches, called diverticula, are pushed out through the wall of the bowel) and haemorrhoids (piles) – problems we'd all like to avoid. If you don't eat a lot of these wholefoods, chances are you're not getting enough fibre. You're not alone; most people only get about half the recommended levels, one in five people over 65 suffer from constipation.

Not only is fibre important for the health of your bowel, it can also be good for your heart. Studies have shown that eating plenty of soluble fibre found in fruit, vegetables and oats can reduce your levels of LDL – low-density lipoprotein. This is called 'bad' cholesterol, because it helps make plaque deposits that line your arteries and can lead to heart attacks and stroke.

Fibre in your diet can help in managing type 2 diabetes, as it helps to slow the rise in blood sugar after you eat and so can lower your risk of being overweight. It also helps you feel full, so you eat less.

There are two main types of fibre: insoluble and soluble. Most plant foods contain a mixture of the two. Insoluble fibre is the tough fibrous part of the plant. You'll find it in wholegrain foods, such as wholegrain bread, wholegrain breakfast cereals, wholewheat pasta and wholegrain (brown) rice. Soluble fibre is found mostly in beans, lentils, oats, fruit and vegetables.

Both types of fibre have numerous health benefits. The insoluble kind is really important for helping your gut work properly, encouraging the natural rhythmical movements of the intestines and speeding the passage of food to the bowel.

HOW MUCH FIBRE SHOULD YOU EAT?

You should be eating about 30g a day, which is 1½ times more than the current average intake (18g). This will be quite a tall order for most people, but according to government guidelines it will help reduce the risk of heart disease, type 2 diabetes and bowel cancer. Here are some ways to reach your target:

✓ Include beans and lentils in your meals at least once a week, and then gradually increase to twice weekly or more. Make a simple dahl (see Lentil and Vegetable Dahl with Cashew Nuts, page 198), add a tin of lentils to vegetable soup (see Easy Vegetable Soup, page 199), or make a healthy salad with mixed beans (try Warm Halloumi Salad, page 195). Combine a tin of red kidney beans with leftover pasta and tinned sweetcorn for a super-quick meal, or add a tin of beans in place of half the meat to bolognese, chilli and shepherd's pie.

✓ Aim for at least five portions of fruit and vegetables a day, ideally seven (see page 71). Have fresh fruit for snacks instead of biscuits or crisps, and include at least two vegetables with each main meal.

✓ Start the day with a bowl of porridge (see Berry Porridge, page 166 and Cinnamon Porridge with Banana and Nuts, page 167) or breakfast cereals labelled wholegrain, for example bran flakes, muesli or Weetabix. If you find them boring, you can jazz them up by adding sliced strawberries, or scatter over some flaked almonds or hazelnuts.

✓ Swap white bread (which is low in fibre) for wholegrain breads, such as wholemeal, rye or oatmeal (which contain more than twice as much B vitamins and iron, and treble the fibre).

✓ Use wholegrains, such as barley in vegetable stews and bulgur wheat in casseroles or stir-fries. Make a wholegrain pilaf (rice dish cooked in a seasoned broth) with a mixture of barley, wild rice, brown rice, stock and herbs.

THE GOOD GUYS

Here are some everyday foods that provide lots of fibre:

Wholegrain breakfast cereals
All-Bran
Fruit & Fibre
bran flakes
Shredded Wheat
muesli (no added sugar)
Weetabix
porridge oats
Wholegrain breads
wholemeal bread
rye bread

oatmeal bread
seeded bread

Grains

wholewheat pasta
brown rice
bulgur wheat
barley
quinoa (strictly speaking this is a seed, pronounced keen-wah)

Fresh fruit

apples, pears
strawberries, raspberries, blackberries, blueberries
oranges, satsumas, clementines
bananas
peaches, apricots, nectarines

Vegetables

carrots, butternut squash
broccoli, spinach, cabbage, kale
potatoes, parsnips, sweet potatoes
green beans

Pulses

red kidney beans
butter beans
chickpeas
baked beans
red, puy and green lentils

Nuts and seeds

peanuts, almonds, Brazil nuts, hazelnuts, cashews and pistachios
sunflower, sesame, pumpkin and chia seeds

Protein

You'll find protein in meat, fish, poultry, eggs, milk, cheese and yogurt as well as plant-derived foods like tofu, Quorn, beans, lentils, nuts, seeds, bread, pasta and rice. Protein is needed for building, maintaining and repairing all body cells, including muscle, skin, hair and organs. It also needed for making enzymes, hormones and antibodies.

Although you are no longer growing, protein is still important as you get older. It will preserve your muscle strength and reduce muscle loss (two key features of the ageing process), boost your resistance to stress, anxiety and depression, and even help you to think more clearly.

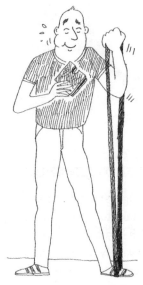

Until recently, scientists believed that the protein requirement decreased with age because most people tend to lose 0.5–2 per cent of their muscle mass per year after the age of about fifty (although it can begin in your forties and will accelerate in your sixties and beyond). This age-related loss of muscle is called *sarcopenia*. Symptoms include loss of strength and poor balance. Caused by lack of exercise and poor nutrition, it can dramatically reduce your ability to perform everyday activities, affect your general mobility and your quality of life unless specific measures are taken to prevent it. However, new findings suggest that eating *more* protein can help offset this age-related muscle loss. Combine this with weight bearing exercise, such as walking, and resistance training exercises, such as push-ups, resistance band or dumb-bell exercises at least twice a week and you can prevent muscle loss, build strength and even reverse the process completely. For a detailed description of these exercises, see *Sod Sixty!* and *Sod Seventy!* In other words, use it or lose it.

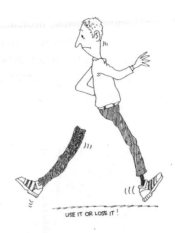

USE IT OR LOSE IT !

HOW MUCH PROTEIN SHOULD YOU EAT?

The latest evidence suggests that people over sixty should aim to up their protein intake to *more* than that recommended for younger adults (which is 50g a day). You can get all the protein you need by eating a variety of foods from both animal sources (meat, fish, poultry, eggs, milk, cheese and plain yogurt), and plant sources (rice, pasta, tofu, Quorn, beans, lentils, nuts and seeds). You should try to eat a variety of protein foods as each contains different amino acids (the building blocks of protein). This way, low levels of a particular amino acid in one food will be balanced by higher levels in another, for example, lentils with rice or tofu with noodles.

It's a sensible idea to include protein in every meal, as that will ensure it is distributed evenly throughout the day. In practice this means including milk, yogurt or eggs with breakfast; meat, poultry, fish, beans or lentils with your lunch and dinner; and having yogurt or nuts for snacks.

Another reason to eat a wide variety of animal and plant proteins is to obtain a wider range of other nutrients such as fibre, vitamins, minerals and carbohydrate. For example, milk gives you calcium and oily fish gives you omega-3s.

Can protein help weight loss?

Protein helps you feel fuller for longer, and that's good news for anyone wanting to lose weight. Protein-rich foods can reduce hunger, curb cravings and control your appetite, all of which should result in a lower calorie intake. In one study, people who ate eggs for breakfast felt less hungry and consumed fewer calories at subsequent meals than those who ate a breakfast of croissants or sugary cereal.

However, this doesn't mean you need to follow a 'high protein' diet – these diets usually contain lots of meat and fat, and little fibre and carbohydrate. Eating this way can make you feel tired, make you constipated and cause nutritional imbalances. What's more, high protein diets are usually hard to stick to week in week out, and there is no evidence that they 'work' any better than other type of diet. Instead, simply include protein in each meal, such as Mediterranean Fish Stew (page 182), Chicken Tagine (page 179) or Tofu and Red Pepper Stir-Fry (page 190) and snack on protein-rich foods such as yogurt, milk and nuts instead of biscuits and cakes.

Is too much protein harmful?

For most people, eating more protein than you need isn't harmful but it isn't beneficial either. It won't make you stronger or build bigger muscles. Excess protein is broken down into urea (which is excreted by the body in your urine) and fuel, which is either used for energy or stored as fat if your calorie intake exceeds your output.

However, if you have a kidney condition, you must avoid excessive protein and should follow the advice of your doctor or registered dietitian about your diet.

THE GOOD GUYS

Here are some everyday foods that provide protein:

Red and white meat
  lean beef, pork, lamb
  chicken and turkey
Fish
  oily fish (salmon, trout, pilchards, herring, sardines)
  white fish (haddock, cod, plaice)

Dairy products
> milk
> cheese
> yogurt (plain is best, sweeten with fresh fruit or a little honey)
> eggs

Nuts and seeds
> peanuts, almonds, cashews and Brazil nuts
> sunflower, pumpkin, sesame and chia seeds

Beans and lentils
> red kidney, butter and cannellini beans
> red, brown and green lentils
> baked beans
> chickpeas

Soya and Quorn products
> soya milk alternative
> tofu
> Quorn

Grains and cereals (contain smaller but useful amounts of protein)
> wholemeal bread
> wholegrain rice
> wholegrain pasta

Water

Water might not seem like an essential nutrient, but it is crucial for good health. It makes up 60 per cent of our body weight. Water helps regulate your temperature, gets rid of waste and allows you to absorb and transport nutrients around the body.

As we get older, we can become more prone to dehydration because our bodies lose the ability to regulate fluid levels and our sense of thirst may not be as sharp. Certain medicines (such as diuretics) also increase the risk of becoming dehydrated. Water is especially important if you are increasing the fibre in your diet, since fibre absorbs water.

Dehydration can make you feel tired and lethargic, and can cause headaches, dizziness and a loss of concentration. Two early signs of dehydration are thirst and dark coloured urine. Not drinking enough is one of the most common causes of constipation. In the long term, it can increase the risk of heart disease, infection and falls. One sign that you're drinking enough is the colour of your urine. It should be pale yellow. If it is bright or dark yellow, you need to drink more.

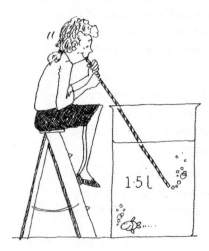

HOW MUCH SHOULD YOU DRINK?

Exactly how much you need to drink depends on several things, including the weather and how active you are, but as a rough guide go with the recommendation from the Department of Health of 6–8 glasses of fluid each day, that's about 1.2–1.5 litres.

Plain old water is perfect but tea and coffee, herb and fruit teas, milk, hot chocolate, low calorie soft drinks and fruit juices also count towards your daily fluid target. Tea, coffee and other drinks containing caffeine will have a slight diuretic effect (meaning they make you go to the loo more often) but do not dehydrate you as once thought. *These drinks still help you stay hydrated.*

To get your quota in, schedule a drink during the times of the day when you already have a routine, such as upon waking, mid-morning, with lunch, mid-afternoon tea and with your evening meal.

If you don't like plain water, try infusing it with a slice of lemon or lime, a few raspberries (or watermelon) or some fresh mint leaves.

Use an App such as iDrinkWater or Daily Water (both free from your app store) to track, store and analyse your intake as well as give you water drinking reminders.

Keep an eye on how much alcohol you drink. Alcohol is a stronger diuretic, and drinks with a high proportion of alcohol, such as spirits, will increase your fluid loss, and add to the effect you feel the next morning, as dehydration is part of the cause of hangover symptoms.

Some people may need to have their amount of fluids restricted due to medical reasons such as kidney or liver disease. Check with your doctor about a suitable fluid intake level for you.

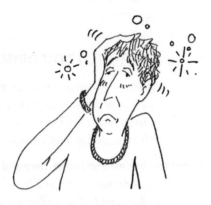

SHOULD I DRINK... MINERAL WATER OR TAP WATER?

Mineral water contains small amounts of minerals, but not enough to make a significant contribution to your diet. Tap water is no less 'pure' and no worse for you than bottled mineral water.

Is it possible to drink too much water?

Taking in too much fluid is rare but can be harmful. Drinking more than 4 litres over a short time can upset the body's sodium balance, and cause a potentially fatal condition called hyponatraemia, or water intoxication. This can cause dizziness, nausea, bloating, lapses in consciousness and seizures due to swelling of the brain. However, it's fairly difficult to over-drink – you'll feel uncomfortably full and bloated long before you reach the danger zone – so you probably don't need to worry about it. Drinking too little is a far greater concern for most people.

Vitamins and minerals

Vitamins support the immune system, help the brain function properly and help convert food into energy. They are important for healthy skin and hair, controlling growth and balancing hormones. Some vitamins – the B vitamins and vitamin C – must be provided by your daily diet, as they cannot be stored in your body.

Minerals are needed for structural and regulatory functions, including bone strength, haemoglobin manufacture, fluid balance and muscle contraction.

Several key vitamins and minerals may be in short supply as you get older. According to the latest National Diet and Nutrition Survey, one in ten older people have deficient intakes of vitamin B12, folate, calcium, vitamin D, potassium, magnesium and iron. Here's an easy-to-follow guide to the whys and wherefores of these essential nutrients:

Vitamin A

Vitamin A is needed to help your immune system work properly, enable vision in dim light and keep your skin and the linings of the respiratory tract and digestive system healthy. It also helps to keep the skin healthy.

Daily intake: 700 micrograms (mcg) for men; 600 mcg for women.

How to get your daily intake: It's found in eggs, cheese, oily fish (such as sardines, mackerel and salmon), whole milk and yogurt, and margarine (which is fortified by law). Liver is the most concentrated source of vitamin A but you shouldn't eat it more than once a week. You can also get your vitamin A from foods rich in beta-carotene, which is converted into vitamin A in the body. The best sources of beta-carotene are orange and red fruit and vegetables (such as carrots, red peppers, butternut squash, apricots and mangoes) as well as leafy green vegetables (such as spinach and watercress).

Thiamin (vitamin B1)

Thiamin works with the other B vitamins to convert carbohydrate, fat and protein into energy. It also helps keep the nervous system healthy.

Daily intake: 1 milligram (mg) a day for men; 0.8mg a day for women.

How to get your daily intake: It's found in a wide range of foods, including nuts, wholegrain bread, pasta and rice, oats, eggs, liver, vegetables and fruit.

Riboflavin (vitamin B2)

Like thiamin, riboflavin helps convert carbohydrate, fat and protein into energy. It is also needed for healthy skin, eyes and the proper functioning of the nervous system.

Daily intake: 1.3 milligrams (mg) a day for men; 1.1mg a day for women.

How to get your daily intake: The best sources of riboflavin are milk, yogurt, cheese and eggs. Smaller amounts are also found in wholegrain bread, brown rice and breakfast cereals (that are fortified). It is destroyed by ultraviolet light so make sure you keep these foods out of direct sunlight.

Niacin (vitamin B3)

Niacin also helps convert carbohydrate, fat and protein into energy, as well as helping keep the nervous system, digestive system and skin healthy.

Daily intake: 17 milligrams (mg) a day for men; 13mg a day for women.

How to get your daily intake: Niacin is found in meat, fish, poultry, bread, potatoes, eggs and milk.

Pyridoxine (vitamin B6)

This works with the other B vitamins to convert carbohydrate, fat and protein into energy. It also helps make red blood cells and keep the immune system healthy.

Daily intake: 1.4 milligrams (mg) a day for men; 1.2mg a day for women.

How to get your daily intake: Vitamin B6 is found in many foods including wholegrain bread, brown rice and oats, meat, poultry, fish, eggs, vegetables, milk and nuts.

Vitamin B12

Vitamin B12 is important for making red blood cells and DNA, and for the proper functioning of the nervous system. It also acts with folic acid and vitamin B6 to control homocysteine levels. High levels of homocysteine are associated with an increased risk of heart disease, stroke and dementia. Consuming too little can result in fatigue, depression, anaemia (abnormal red blood cell development and shortness of breath) and nerve damage.

Daily intake: 1.5 micrograms (mcg).

How to get your daily intake: The richest sources include fish, meat, poultry, eggs, milk and milk products. For vegans, the Vegetarian Society recommends a multi-vitamin and mineral supplement that provides 10mcg of B12.

Folate

Folate works with B12 in the formation of red blood cells and for the growth and reproduction of cells. Too little of this essential

B vitamin may contribute to pernicious anaemia, which results in tiredness, apathy and depression.

Daily intake: 200 micrograms (mcg).

How to get your daily intake: Vegetables, especially dark leafy ones like spinach, cabbage and broccoli, fruit, fortified breakfast cereals and bread, yeast extract, nuts and pulses.

Vitamin C

Vitamin C is needed for growth and repair of body cells, and for the formation of connective tissues, red blood cells, and exercise-related hormones, including adrenaline. It also promotes healthy blood vessels and gums and strengthens the immune system. It is a powerful antioxidant, which can protect cell from damage.

Daily intake: 40 milligrams (mg).

How to get your daily intake: The best food sources are fresh fruit and vegetables, particularly citrus fruit, berries and currants, as well as peppers and dark green leafy vegetables such as spinach and cabbage.

Calcium

Calcium is important for building and maintaining strong bones. It also helps with blood clotting, nerve and muscle function. Unfortunately, surveys show that as we age we consume less calcium in our diets. If you don't get enough, it leaches out of your bones and increases the risk of brittle bones (osteoporosis) and fractures.

Daily intake: 700 milligrams (mg).

How to get your daily intake: Try to get three servings of milk, yogurt and cheese a day – these are the richest sources. Other good dietary sources include tinned sardines (and other tinned fish with edible bones), dark green leafy vegetables, almonds, sesame seeds, tofu and dried figs (see page 50).

Vitamin D

Vitamin D is essential for healthy bones and preventing osteoporosis. Recent studies suggest that vitamin D may also protect against several chronic diseases, including heart disease, dementia, bowel cancer and type 2 diabetes, although the exact connection isn't yet clear. In 2012, researchers from the University of Copenhagen found people who had low vitamin D levels had a 64 per cent higher risk of heart attack. Some researchers have linked the lack of sunlight in Scotland to the country's high rates of heart disease.

People who have more vitamin D in the blood are 40 per cent less likely to develop bowel cancer than those with low levels, according to a 2010 study published in the *British Medical Journal*. In one study, women with the highest levels of vitamin D were 50–70 per cent less likely to suffer from breast cancer than those with the lowest levels.

Daily intake: There is no official recommended daily allowance in the UK but the EU advises 5 micrograms (mcg) daily.

How to get your daily intake: Unlike other vitamins, where our intake comes from food, we get around 90 per cent of our vitamin D from the action of sunlight (ultraviolet B rays) on our skin. Unfortunately, this process becomes less efficient as we get older, so it's easy to fall short of this vitamin. The current advice is to spend short spells – 15 minutes a day from April to September – in the sun with face and arms uncovered, without suncream (anything over factor 8 blocks out the ultraviolent light the body needs to create vitamin D) and in the middle of the day. This guidance was drawn up by a group of seven organisations, including Cancer Research UK and the National Osteoporosis Society.

How much vitamin D is produced from sunlight depends on the time of day, where you live in the world and the colour of your skin. The more skin you expose the more vitamin D is produced. People with darker skin will need to spend longer in the sun to produce the same amount of vitamin D. But make sure you always cover up or protect your skin before you start turning red or burn.

During the winter months our skin can't produce enough vitamin D, as the sunlight hasn't got enough UVB radiation. So we have to rely on the body's vitamin D stores and our diet. But it's harder to get the right amount of vitamin D from food. There are only three categories of foods that contain significant amounts of it: eggs, liver and oily fish, such as tuna (tinned in oil), sardines, salmon and mackerel. Vitamin D is found only in the yolk of the egg, so make sure you use the whole egg when making omelettes or scrambled eggs. Two eggs will give you around two thirds of your daily requirement (5mcg). A portion of liver (100g) supplies around one fifth of what you need. Look out also for foods with added vitamin D, which supply useful amounts during the winter months. *You need fat or oil to absorb vitamin D*, so if you're having a vitamin D fortified food such as breakfast cereal, add whole or semi-skimmed (not skimmed) milk. Each of the following provides the recommended daily amount of 5mcg:

- 3 eggs
- ½ tsp (2.5 ml) cod liver oil
- 100g tinned sardines
- 60g mackerel
- 70g salmon
- 170g tinned tuna (in oil)

SHOULD I TAKE VITAMIN D SUPPLEMENTS?

The National Institute for Health and Clinical Excellence (NICE) recommends supplements containing 10mcg (400IU) vitamin D each day for those over 65. Some researchers recommend up to 25mcg daily. If you think you may be at risk of vitamin D deficiency, it's a good idea to talk to the nurse at your health centre or pharmacist.

Vitamin E

Vitamin E is a powerful antioxidant, which works with vitamin C to protect cell membranes from damage. It also helps to maintain healthy skin, eyes and strengthen the immune system.

Daily intake: 4 milligrams (mg) for men; 3mg for women.

How to get your daily intake: The richest food sources are vegetable oils, margarine, wholegrain bread, oily fish, nuts, seeds, avocado, green leafy vegetables and egg yolk.

Potassium

This essential mineral is vital for cell function and, combined with a low salt intake, has also been shown to help reduce high blood pressure and the risk of kidney stones. Unfortunately, surveys show that many older people don't get the recommended 3500mg of potassium a day.

Daily intake: 3500 milligrams (mg).

How to get your daily intake: Fruit and vegetables are by far the richest dietary sources of potassium. Bananas, prunes, oranges, broccoli and potatoes are particularly rich in potassium. By including fruit and vegetables in every meal, you should be able to get enough.

Magnesium

Magnesium plays a crucial role in many different body processes. Getting enough can help keep your immune system working properly, your heart healthy and your bones strong. Many wholefoods, including cereal, fruit and vegetables, contain magnesium. But it is often lost in commercial processing so foods like crisps, shop-bought cakes and biscuits contain very little. Absorption of magnesium decreases with age, which increases your risk of deficiency. Some medications, including diuretics (which are prescribed for lowering high blood pressure), may also reduce magnesium absorption.

Daily intake: 300 milligrams (mg) for men, 270mg for women.

How to get your daily intake: Eating mostly unprocessed and plant-based foods, including fresh fruit, vegetables, nuts, whole grains, beans and seeds, is the best way to get enough magnesium.

Iron

Iron is essential for the formation of haemoglobin, the oxygen-carrying pigment in red blood cells. It is also needed for a healthy immune system and preventing iron deficiency anaemia, which can leave you feeling tired and fatigued.

Daily intake: 8.7 milligrams (mg) for men and post-menopausal women; 14.8mg for pre-menopausal women.

How to get your daily intake: Include iron-rich foods in your diet. Meat and offal are the richest sources but there are plenty of vegetarian sources, such as wholegrains, beans, lentils, green leafy vegetables, dried fruit, nuts, seeds, tofu, egg yolk and fortified breakfast cereals. However, 'non-haem' iron in plant foods is less readily absorbed than 'haem' iron in animal products (meat and fish). You can increase your uptake of iron by eating these foods with a source of vitamin C (e.g. fruit or vegetables).

SHOULD I TAKE IRON SUPPLEMENTS?

If you are feeling very tired, you may have anaemia and should talk to your doctor. A simple test can determine your iron level and if iron deficiency is diagnosed, your doctor will recommend supplements. These may be taken in liquid or pill form. The usual recommended dose is 60–100 milligrams (mg) per day for three months. However, if you are not deficient then you shouldn't take supplements – they may do more harm than good.

Zinc

Zinc is crucial to the activity of more than seventy enzymes involved in the metabolism of proteins, fats and carbohydrates. It also helps heal wounds and promote recovery from soft tissue injuries, as well as keeping the immune system healthy and fighting infection.

Daily intake: 7 milligrams (mg).

How to get your daily intake: Zinc is found in nuts, lentils, beans, eggs, wholegrain cereals, meat, milk and dairy products.

Selenium

Selenium acts as an antioxidant that helps protect cells against damage from free radicals (see page 69) as well as heart disease and cancer.

Daily intake: 55 micrograms (mcg).

How to get your daily intake: Best sources are nuts, especially Brazil nuts, wholegrain bread, pasta and rice, fish (especially prawns) and eggs.

Sodium

Chemically salt is sodium chloride, made up of one molecule of sodium (roughly 40 per cent) and one molecule of chloride (roughly 60 per cent). While it is essential for fluid balance, nerve transmission, muscle function, digestion and blood pressure, it is possible to consume too much.

Daily intake: A minimum of 575 milligrams (mg) of sodium – equivalent to 1.4 grams (g) of salt – is needed, but you should have no more than 2.4g sodium (6g salt).

How to get your daily intake: Sodium is found in all foods but high quantities are found in processed foods such as ready meals, pizza, ham, bacon, sausages, burgers, fast food, sauces, soup and breakfast cereals.

SHOULD I TAKE VITAMIN SUPPLEMENTS?

With the right food choices, you should be able to get all the vitamins and minerals you need to keep healthy and ward off diseases. There is solid evidence that diets rich in vitamins and minerals, and antioxidants in particular, lessen the risks of heart disease and cancer. But, despite their popularity, there's scant proof that vitamins in pills give the same benefits as food.

A comprehensive review of 26 studies concluded that for healthy people without nutritional deficiencies, there's little benefit to be gained by taking multivitamins. Similarly, a long-term clinical trial over 14,000 adults aged fifty plus found that those who took daily multivitamins were no less likely to suffer from heart disease, stroke or cognitive decline than non-users. There's little evidence either for vitamin C supplements – they won't stop you catching a cold. More worrying is the fact that high doses of vitamin A, vitamin E and beta-carotene supplements have been associated with an increased risk of cancer. Calcium and iron supplements are not recommended unless advised by your doctor.

However, a vitamin D supplement *is* recommended for those over 65 (see page 151) as well as those with dark skin or limited sun exposure. The best advice is food first, supplements second – and only if genuinely needed. In a nutshell: while multivitamins are generally harmless, there's no guarantee that they will help you live longer or reduce your risk of disease.

SUMMARY OF VITAMINS AND MINERALS

Vitamin	Needed for	Best food and other sources
A	Vision in dim light; healthy skin and linings of the digestive tract, nose and throat	Full fat dairy products, meat, offal, oily fish, margarine
Beta-carotene	Antioxidant, which protects against certain cancers; converts into vitamin A	Fruit and vegetables e.g. apricots, peppers, tomatoes, mangoes, broccoli, squash, carrots, watercress
Vitamin B1 (thiamine)	Releases energy from carbohydrates; healthy nerves and digestive system	Wholemeal bread and cereals, pulses, meat, sunflower seeds

Vitamin B2 (riboflavin)	Releases energy from carbohydrates; healthy skin, eyes and nerves	Milk and dairy products, meat, eggs, soya products
Vitamin B3 (niacin)	Releases energy from carbohydrates; healthy skin, nerves and digestion	Meat and offal, nuts, milk and dairy products, eggs, wholegrain cereals
Vitamin B6 (pyridoxine)	Metabolism of protein, carbohydrate, fat; red blood cell manufacture; healthy immune system	Pulses, nuts, eggs, cereals, fish, bananas
Folic acid	Formation of DNA and red blood cells; reduces risk of spina bifida in developing babies	Green leafy vegetables, yeast extract, pulses, nuts, citrus fruit
Vitamin B12	Formation of red blood cells; energy metabolism	Milk and dairy products, meat; fish, fortified breakfast cereals, soya products and yeast extract
Vitamin C	Healthy connective tissue, bones, teeth, blood vessels, gums and teeth; promotes immune function; helps iron absorption	Fruit and vegetables e.g. raspberries, blackcurrants, kiwi, oranges, peppers, broccoli, cabbage, tomatoes
Vitamin D	Builds strong bones; needed to absorb calcium and phosphorus	Sunlight, oily fish, fortified margarine and breakfast cereals, eggs
Vitamin E	Antioxidant, which helps protect against heart disease; promotes normal cell growth and development	Vegetable oils, oily fish, nuts, seeds, egg yolk, avocado

Mineral	Needed for	Best food sources
Calcium	Builds bone and teeth; blood clotting; nerve and muscle function	Milk and dairy products, sardines, dark green leafy vegetables, pulses, Brazil nuts, almonds, figs, sesame seeds
Iron	Formation of red blood cells; oxygen transport; prevents anaemia	Meat and offal, wholegrain cereals, fortified breakfast cereals, pulses, green leafy vegetables, nuts, sesame and pumpkin seeds

Zinc	Healthy immune system; wound healing; skin; cell growth	Eggs, wholegrain cereals, meat, nuts and seeds
Magnesium	Healthy bones; muscle and nerve function; cell formation	Cereals, fruit, vegetables, milk, nuts and seeds
Potassium	Fluid balance; muscle and nerve function	Fruit, vegetables, cereals, nuts and seeds
Sodium	Fluid balance; muscle and nerve function	Salt, processed meat, ready meals, sauces, soup, cheese, bread
Selenium	Antioxidant, which helps protect against heart disease and cancer	Cereals, vegetables, dairy products, meat, eggs, nuts and seeds

Salt

We need a little bit of salt to keep healthy but eating too much leads to raised blood pressure. The reason we need some salt is to help regulate the volume of blood circulating in the body and the movement of fluid between cells. It also helps cells to take in nutrients from the blood and helps muscles contract. But the fact is most of us consume more salt than we need for good health.

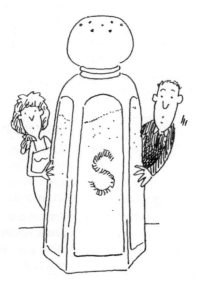

HOW MUCH SALT SHOULD YOU CONSUME?

We need a lot less than most people imagine – just 1.4g a day is all that's actually needed. But, on average, we eat a whopping 8.1g a day. Currently, the Department of Health and most other medical organisations recommend limiting your daily salt intake to 6g.

Why is too much salt bad for you?

If you eat more salt than you need then the volume of body fluid increases and pushes up your blood pressure. In most people, this is only temporary and your blood pressure will return to normal as the excess salt and fluid are excreted in your urine. However, some people are more sensitive to salt than others and generally as we get older, our sensitivity to salt increases. This means excess salt may cause an above-normal rise in blood pressure. To reduce your risk of developing high blood pressure, you should cut down on salty foods. As 75 per cent of the salt we eat comes from everyday processed food, this means limiting foods like ready meals, sauces, dressings, bacon, ham and crisps.

Check the nutritional information on food labels. Nowadays many show the salt content as a percentage of the Reference Intake (RI) (see page 56) or have colour-coded nutrition information to show whether the food is high (red), medium (amber) or low (green) in salt. As a guide when considering foods in the supermarket:

- a high amount of salt is more than 1.5g per 100g (600mg sodium)
- a low amount of salt is 0.3g per 100g (100mg sodium)

High blood pressure increases the risk of heart disease and stroke. Excess salt also leaches calcium from the bones, making them weaker, aggravates asthma, puts stress on the kidneys and may increase the risk of stomach cancer. Populations with a high average salt intake have a higher average blood pressure and higher levels of hypertension (high blood pressure) than others.

HOW MUCH SALT ARE YOU EATING?

Food	Salt (in grams)
Bran flakes (30g)	0.3
Beef lasagne ready meal (400g)	1.7
Crisps (1 small bag, 32.5g)	0.4
Wholemeal bread (1 slice)	0.5
Pasta sauce (100g)	1.0
Tomato ketchup (15g)	0.3
Pork sausage (one, 50g)	1.1
Bacon (2 rashers, 40g)	1.2
Ham (1 slice, 20g)	0.4
Pizza (half, 200g)	2.5

How to cut down on salt

- taste food before adding extra salt during cooking or at the table
- use herbs and spices such as garlic, oregano and lemon juice to add flavour to meals instead of some of the salt you would normally add
- choose reduced or 'no added' salt versions of tinned foods, such as baked beans and lentils
- eat less processed foods: burgers, sausages, chicken nuggets, pasta sauces, ready meals, crisps, pizza, bought sandwiches, ketchup, dressings and breakfast cereals
- limit high salt foods: ham, bacon, smoked meat and fish, prawns, soy sauce and stock cubes
- swap salty snacks like crisps for fresh fruit, unsalted nuts or plain popcorn
- limit ready meals, takeaways and fast foods

Alcohol

The health effects of alcohol have been debated for many years, and some doctors are reluctant to encourage alcohol consumption because of the health consequences of excessive drinking. However, in some research studies alcohol *in moderation* (no more than one drink (unit) a day for women and two for men) – has been associated with a reduced risk of heart disease in people over 45. Studies show that compared with people who drink no alcohol, those who have one drink a day are 14–25 per cent less likely to have heart disease or stroke. That's because *a small amount* of alcohol increases levels of HDL cholesterol, the type that's good for your heart. It can also help stop platelets sticking together and forming blood clots ('thrombosis') and causing a heart attack. But don't take it as an excuse to over-indulge – drinking more than that does not offer any extra benefit.

In fact, alcohol increases the risk of five common cancers, including mouth and throat, bowel and breast cancer. The World Cancer Research Fund advises that you avoid drinking alcohol as much as possible to help prevent cancer – aim for no more than two drinks a day if you're a man and one drink a day if you're a woman. As a rough guide, a drink (1 unit) contains 10–15g of pure alcohol, which is equivalent to:

- half a pint of normal strength beer, lager or cider
- one 25ml measure of spirits such as vodka or whisky
- half a standard (175ml) glass of wine

However, many alcoholic drinks are stronger than we realise (for example, most wine these days contains 12–13 per cent alcohol; previously it contained around 8 per cent) and serving sizes are also bigger than they used to be. For example, a standard glass of wine has increased from 125ml before the 1990s to 175ml or even 250ml nowadays. If you enjoy a drink at home, check the amount you pour into your glass – you may find it's more than you thought.

The NHS advises a *maximum* of four units daily and 21 units weekly for men; three units a day and 14 units a week for women. You shouldn't drink more than this as it can dramatically push up your risk of liver disease, high blood pressure, stroke, heart disease and cancer. Drinking a large amount in one go (binge drinking) is especially harmful and can damage the brain.

If you're trying to lose weight, though, even moderate drinking could sabotage your efforts. A glass of wine, for example, clocks up the same number of calories as one ice cream cone, while a pint of lager is equal to a doughnut. Sharing a bottle of wine with your partner not only exceeds daily unit guidelines but is the calorie equivalent of eating two slices of cake.

While research and the debate about the health benefits of alcohol continue, the key seems to be moderation. Drink too much and you can damage your body, but in moderation – one drink a day for women and two a day for men – you might enjoy alcohol's health benefits.

ALCOHOL AND FOOD EQUIVALENTS

Type of alcohol	Amount (in units)	Food equivalent
1 small glass champagne	1 unit	1 chocolate digestive biscuit
1 glass sherry	1 unit	1 sausage
1 large gin & tonic	2 units	1 slice of cake
1 pint normal strength beer, lager or cider	2 units	1 doughnut
1 standard glass wine	2 units	1 bag of crisps
2 bottles of beer	3½ units	½ pizza

Is red wine good for you?

Red wine may have heart health benefits thanks to its high content of antioxidants. Scientists have found that red wines have higher levels of antioxidant compounds called polyphenols, which come from the coloured skins of grapes, so red wine tends to have a greater concentration of polyphenols than white wine. In general, the darker the wine the higher the antioxidant content. In tests cabernet sauvignon grapes were shown to contain the most, followed by merlot, zinfandel, syrah and petit syrah. But don't use this an excuse to over-indulge – having more than one or two drinks a day will harm, not benefit, your health.

How to read food labels

Food labels provide lots of information that can help you achieve a healthy diet but are often confusing – it can sometimes feel like you need a science or nutrition degree to decode them. But fear not, here's how to decipher them:

1. Begin by reading the list of ingredients
The ingredients are listed in descending order of weight, i.e. the most to the least. This means that the first few ingredients make up the bulk of the product. By law, if an ingredient is mentioned in the name of a food, e.g. in 'apple pie', or is shown on the label, the amount of that ingredient contained in the food (e.g. apple) must be given as a percentage.

2. Read the nutrition label on the back of the packaging
This label includes the following nutrients per 100g or per 100ml and sometimes per portion of food:

Energy (kJ/kcals)
Fat (g)
Saturates (saturated fat) (g)
Carbohydrate (g)
Sugars (g)
Protein (g)
Salt (g)

Should they want to, food manufacturers can include additional nutritional information. If however, a food product makes a health claim for a specific nutrient, then the nutritional information for that nutrient *must* be listed. For example, if a food is described as high in vitamin C, the vitamin C content must be listed within the nutritional information.

3. Read the nutrition labels on the front of the packaging
Front of pack labels give you an at-a-glance guide to the product's energy, fat, saturated fat, sugar and salt content *per portion* and the contribution each nutrient makes towards the Reference Intake (RI)*. This is usually in a colour-coded format to help you make a quick assessment of the product's overall nutritional value. Just bear in mind that a manufacturer's idea of a portion may be different from yours.

* Reference Intakes (RIs) are a guide to how much energy and key nutrients the average person needs in order to have a healthy

diet. They are not targets, rather a very simple approximation of your nutritional needs. The RIs are based on a 2000-calorie diet (they don't differentiate between men and women or allow for different ages or activity levels).

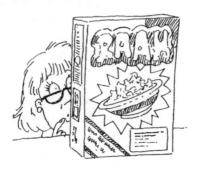

These are the Reference Intakes (RIs) listed on food labels:

Energy	2000kcal (8400kJ)
Total fat	70g
Of which saturates	20g
Total sugars*	90g
Salt	6g

* Total sugars include sugars occurring naturally in foods as well as added sugars.

Red, amber and green colour coding

This is the Food Standards Agency-approved labelling system, which was first introduced in 2007, and tells you whether the food contains high, medium or low amounts of each of the above nutrients in 100g of the food. Since 2013, food manufacturers must by law use a standardised combination of nutrition information and colour coding to show how much fat, salt and sugar and how many calories are in each product. It's an easy-to-use traffic like system:

Green means low
Amber means medium
Red means high

Many foods will have a mixture of red, amber and greens. The idea is, when you're choosing between similar products, to go for more greens and ambers, and fewer reds.

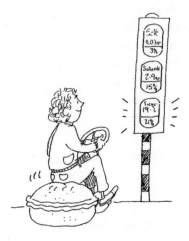

As a rule of thumb, the more green on the label, the healthier choice, although this doesn't strictly apply to all products. Foods such as olive oil, nuts and cheese are coded red for their high fat content but this disguises the fact they are rich in other nutrients, such as monounsaturated fats in olive oil, vitamin E in nuts or protein in cheese.

The table below shows the general rules of the traffic light system on food labels:

All measures per 100g	Green	Amber	Red
Fat	3g or less	>3g – ≤ 17.5g	More than 17.5g or >21g/portion
Saturated fat	1.5g or less	>1.5g – ≤ 5g	More than 5g or >6g/portion
Sugars	5g or less	>5g – ≤ 22.5g	More than 22.5g or >27g/portion
Salt	0.3g or less	>0.3g – ≤ 1.5g	More than 1.5g or >1.8g/portion

Beware of misleading health claims

A general rule is to treat claims on food labels with caution. 'Low fat', 'no added sugar' and 'all natural' are just some of the terms we see on food packages every day that can lull you into thinking the products are healthier than they actually are. Although some of the terms are defined by law (e.g. 'low fat' means the food must contain no more than 3g of fat per 100g), they can also be misleading. That's because they are often slapped on a food that may not be healthy at all. For example, a breakfast cereal could claim to be low in fat, but could also be high in sugar. Biscuits and cereal bars can claim to be 'reduced fat' but, thanks to their higher content of sugar, may still contain the same number of calories as other similar versions or brands. You'll also see terms like 'all natural' or 'lite' on food packets but *these have no legal definition* – they are simply applied by the manufacturer to make the product look healthier. And be wary of 'no added sugar' foods – these may still contain added ingredients like fruit juice concentrate, rice syrup and agave syrup, which are all sugar.

The best way to decide whether a food is good enough for you is to look at the label. As a rule of thumb, if the product contains more ingredients than you would use to make the equivalent home-made version (especially if some of them are unpronounceable), then don't buy it. Stick to 'real' foods!

Summary of What to Eat

- Adjust your food intake to avoid putting on weight. As a rough guide, the average man over 60 needs about 2000 calories a day, the average woman about 1600.
- A *moderate fat* diet (such as the Mediterranean diet, see Chapter 2) is better for you than a *low fat* diet.
- Swap some of the *saturated fats* (meat, butter) in your diet for *unsaturated fats* (olive oil, oily fish and nuts).
- Snack on *'real' foods*, like fruit, nuts and plain yogurt instead of *processed snacks*, such as biscuits, chocolate and crisps.
- *Carbohydrate* foods, like potatoes, bread, pasta, rice, oats, beans, lentils and fruit should make up about *half* of your

daily calories. Choose wholegrain varieties of bread and cereals wherever possible.

- Eat less *sugar*. Aim to get no more than 5 per cent of your daily calories from 'added' sugar, that's 25g or 6 teaspoons – equivalent to one cupcake or a small bar of chocolate.
- Avoid *sweetened drinks* and eat whole fruit rather than drink fruit juice.
- *Fibre* can prevent many chronic diseases. We need 30g a day – most people get just 18g – from porridge, wholegrain bread and pasta, beans, chickpeas, lentils, fruits and vegetables.
- Getting enough *protein* is especially important as we get older to stave off muscle wasting. Include a portion of meat, fish, dairy products, pulses or eggs in every meal.
- *Vitamin supplements* are unnecessary – with the right food choices, you should be able to get all the vitamins and minerals you need to keep healthy. The exception is vitamin D – a supplement is recommended for the over 65s.
- Getting enough *water* is crucial for good health – drink 6–8 cups or glasses of fluid a day, more in warm weather.
- Too much *salt* may raise blood pressure. Cut back on processed foods: burgers, sausages, ham, bacon, pasta sauces, ready meals, crisps, pizza, bought sandwiches, ketchup, dressings and breakfast cereals.
- Stick to safe *alcohol* limits: four units a day and 21 units a week for men, three units a day and 14 units a week for women.

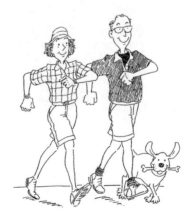

2

EATING THE MEDITERRANEAN WAY

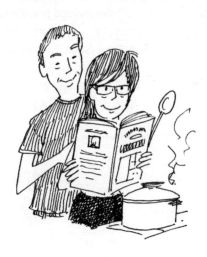

In the last chapter, we learned about the main pillars of a healthy diet and how much of the various nutrients we should be eating to stave off ill health. We also looked at the hazards of eating too much of certain things, like sugar and salt, and discovered that we should be eating a lot more fibre, drinking plenty of water and not too much alcohol. But how does this translate into our day-to-day eating? Exactly how much of all the different foods should we be putting on our plates? What combination of foods should we be aiming at to live a healthier and longer life?

Perhaps the best clues come from studies of the world's healthiest people. They live in countries bordering the Mediterranean Sea and also in the so-called 'Blue Zones'. These are regions, first identified by longevity expert and National Geographic explorer Dan Buettner, where people live extraordinarily long, healthy and happy lives: Sardinia; Okinawa in Japan; Ikaria in Greece; the Nicoya peninsula of Costa Rica and Loma Linda in Southern California. Here, people live, on average, ten years longer than the rest of us. In one Sardinian village there are six centenarians out of 3000 people, as compared to most of America where there's just one centenarian for every 5000 people.

If you look at their habits, you'll find they have several things in common. They enjoy physical activity incorporated naturally into their daily lives (like gardening or walking); a sense of purpose (like caring for grandchildren or doing voluntary work); low stress levels and a slower pace of life; strong family and community connections and a diet characterised by moderate calorific intake, mostly from plant sources.

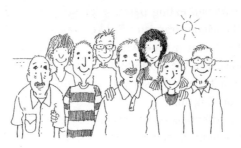

What we can learn from them is that following a mainly plant-based diet, coupled with a healthy amount of exercise, can lead to a much better quality as well as a longer life. They eat very few processed foods; very little meat and they don't overeat. Emphasis is placed on basing every meal on fruit and vegetables, wholegrains, beans, fish, nuts and olive oil.

The latest research suggests that this eating pattern can protect against chronic disease, such as heart attack, stroke, cancer, type 2 diabetes and dementia, thus making you feel better and helping you live longer. While you probably get the biggest pay-off by adopting such a diet early in life, making the necessary changes during midlife is good too. In one study, researchers looked at the dietary habits of more than 10,000 women in their fifties and sixties and compared them to how the women fared health-wise 15 years later. Women who followed a healthy diet during middle age were about 40 per cent more likely to live past the age of seventy without chronic illness and without physical or mental problems than those with less-healthy diets. The healthiest women were those who ate more plant-foods, wholegrains, and fish, ate less red and processed meats and had limited alcohol intake. That's typical of a Mediterranean diet, which is also rich in olive oil and nuts.

In this chapter, we explain how you too can enjoy the healthy benefits of the Mediterranean diet. We'll give you a blueprint to follow and guide you through the simple diet changes that really can help add years to your life.

What exactly is the Mediterranean diet?

Although there's no 'set' Mediterranean diet, we're really talking about the *traditional* eating patterns of people living in countries that border the Mediterranean Sea like Greece, Crete and southern Italy, *circa* 1960 – at a time when rates of chronic disease were among the lowest in the world and life expectancy was among the highest. We don't mean the sort of diet eaten by people holidaying in Benidorm or Magaluf.

The key word here is *traditional*. With faster paced lifestyles and modern conveniences many people living in the Mediterranean region no longer eat as they used to and have adopted 'Westernised' eating habits of fast foods and highly processed foods, inactivity and the introduction of sweets in children's diet. Where these 'new' lifestyle practices prevail the rate of obesity, heart disease and cancer has risen.

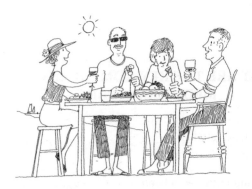

Nutrition experts around the world regard the traditional Mediterranean diet as the gold standard for eating patterns that promote lifelong good health. It is typically defined as one based on food from plant sources: fruit, vegetables, unrefined wholegrains, beans, lentils, nuts, seeds and potatoes. Olive oil is the main source of unsaturated fat, replacing other oils and fats such as margarine and butter. It includes moderate consumption of red wine, fish, dairy, poultry and eggs, and only small amounts of red meat and sugar. The foods eaten are as close to their natural state as possible – fresh, seasonal, unprocessed and flavoured with herbs and spices.

Contrary to popular belief, this diet is not based on huge bowls of pasta. Traditionally, when the Italians eat pasta, it's served in small portions. In fact, typically less than 45 per cent of the calories in a Mediterranean diet come from carbohydrate. Perhaps the best description is that it is not so much a diet as a way of life based around fresh, seasonal food that is unprocessed and eaten with friends and family. One of the most researched diets because of its apparent efficacy, it is now well recognised for its heart-healthy and longevity benefits.

The Mediterranean diet tends to contain a *moderate* amount of fat – it can be up to 40 per cent of total calorie intake – but most of it comes from healthy oils. Scientists say that it is the *type* of fat in your diet rather than the *total amount* that is important when it comes to heart health. A diet rich in olive oil, fish and nuts contains a high proportion of monounsaturated fats and a relatively small amount of saturated fat, which is more beneficial than a diet that's low in fat *per se*.

WHAT ARE THE KEY COMPONENTS OF THE MEDITERRANEAN DIET?

✓ eating primarily plant-based foods, such as fruits and vegetables, wholegrains, legumes (e.g. peas, beans, lentils) and nuts

✓ replacing butter with healthy fats, such as olive oil

✓ using herbs and spices instead of salt to flavour foods

✓ limiting red meat to no more than a few times a month

✓ eating fish and poultry several times a week

✓ drinking wine in moderation (optional)

The diet also recognises the importance of being physically active and enjoying meals with family and friends.

What are the benefits of the Mediterranean Diet?

People who eat a Mediterranean diet have been shown to have a remarkable variety of health benefits, including a lower risk of heart disease, cancer and dementia. These benefits first became clear in the 1950s when scientists discovered that countries in the Mediterranean region had very little heart disease compared with more northerly countries. Since then, the evidence linking a diet based on an abundance of fruit, vegetables, pulses, fish and olive with a reduced risk of heart disease – as well as health and longevity – has been mounting. No other diet has as much documented evidence as the Mediterranean diet. It appears to be a better option than the standard low fat diet for promoting health and preventing chronic disease. Here are six key benefits you can expect from eating the 'Med way':

1. A healthy heart
Research has shown that the traditional Mediterranean diet reduces the risks of heart attack, stroke and deaths from cardiovascular disease. In 2015, scientists from Harokopio University in Athens published results of a study showing that those who adopted a Mediterranean diet were 47 per cent less likely to develop heart disease over a 10-year period than those who didn't.

Encouragingly, you don't need to adopt the whole diet to benefit either. According to their results, the researchers found that each one-point adherence to a Mediterranean style diet (e.g. regular consumption of fish, using olive oil) was associated with a 3 per cent reduction in heart disease risk.

A 2013 study carried out in Spain suggested that a Mediterranean diet is almost as good at reducing the risk of a heart attack as taking statins for people aged 55 to 80. Researchers found that those eating a Mediterranean diet that included extra olive oil or nuts cut their risk of suffering a heart attack or stroke by 30 per cent compared with those following a conventional low fat diet. So convincing were the results that the researchers began following the Mediterranean diet themselves, and after almost five years the trial was stopped as it was considered unethical to allow people to continue eating the low fat regime. People eating the Mediterranean diet also lowered their blood pressure and blood cholesterol and had less inflammation than those eating the low fat diet.

Following the diet has also been shown to reverse the metabolic syndrome, a combination of obesity, high blood pressure and type 2 diabetes that puts you at increased risk of heart disease and stroke.

2. Longer life
A Mediterranean diet can help you live longer. In a 2011 study, researchers compared its effects on longevity in more than a thousand seventy-year-olds over more than forty years. They found that those who ate a Mediterranean diet lived 2–3 years longer than

those who didn't. An analysis of a dozen studies involving more than 1.5 million people published in the *British Medical Journal* found that eating a Mediterranean diet lowers the risk of dying from any cause, including heart disease or stroke by 9 per cent, and reduces the chances of developing cancer, Parkinson's and Alzheimer's disease.

3. Weight loss

Although it's not promoted as a weight loss diet, following a Mediterranean diet can help you shed pounds thanks to its emphasis on high-fibre foods. A 2008 study found that the Mediterranean diet was more effective than a standard low fat diet when it came to weight loss. Volunteers who ate a Mediterranean diet lost an average of 4 kg (9 pounds) in 2 years, whereas those assigned to a low-fat diet lost an average of 3kg (6 pounds) during that time period. Another revealed that, after a year, Mediterranean dieters had managed to keep the weight off, while those following a low fat diet had regained their lost pounds.

4. Less cancer risk

The Mediterranean diet has been shown to provide cancer-preventing benefits. A 2008 analysis published in the *British Medical Journal* showed that following a Mediterranean diet reduced the risk of dying from cancer by 9 per cent. That same year, another study showed that post-menopausal women who followed the Mediterranean diet were 22 per cent less likely to develop breast cancer.

5. Prevent diabetes

There are also benefits for people with type 2 diabetes. A 2009 study by researchers in Italy found that people with type 2 diabetes who followed a Mediterranean diet instead of a standard low fat diet had better blood sugar control and were less likely to need diabetes medication. But it can also help reduce your risk of developing the disease. Another study involving 13,000 people showed that those following a Mediterranean diet were less likely to develop type 2 diabetes. What's more, among those deemed to be at high risk, there was an 83 per cent reduction in the likelihood of developing the disease.

6. Ward off dementia

There is good evidence that eating a Mediterranean diet can reduce the risk of developing problems with memory and thinking, and getting some forms of dementia. One large UK study carried out over thirty years found that men aged between 45 and 59 who followed four or five of the identified lifestyle factors of the diet were found to have a 36 per cent lower risk of developing cognitive decline and a 36 per cent lower risk of developing dementia than those who did not. These factors include taking regular physical exercise, eating a Mediterranean diet, not smoking, preventing or treating diabetes, high blood pressure and obesity and drinking alcohol only in moderation

SIX HEALTHY MEDITERRANEAN-STYLE SNACKS

Swap chocolate and sugary snacks for these protein- and fibre-packed options. These foods stabilise blood sugar levels and satisfy hunger:

1. 1 heaped tablespoon houmous with carrot and celery sticks

2. Oatcakes or rice cakes with peanut butter

3. A couple of squares of plain 70 per cent cocoa solids chocolate

4. A handful of nuts

5. Fresh fruit

6. A pot of plain yogurt

Why does the Mediterranean Diet work?

It is thought that the Mediterranean diet works by lowering inflammation and oxidative stress (cell damage due to free radicals), as well as improving blood sugar control and insulin levels. Fruit and vegetables, whole grains, pulses and nuts are packed with fibre, which slows digestion and helps control blood sugar. The monounsaturated fats in olive oil, nuts and oily fish have powerful anti-inflammatory effects. But the key really lies in the total package of foods, and how the nutrients act together.

WHAT ARE FREE RADICALS?

Free radicals are by-products of normal body processes, such as the conversion of food into energy. When oxygen is metabolised, it creates free radicals, which steal electrons from other molecules, causing damage. The body can cope with some free radicals (and needs them to function effectively) but an overload can trigger the inflammation process that causes clogged arteries, thrombosis, heart disease and cancer.

The Mediterranean Diet Rules

The essence of Mediterranean eating is generous quantities of vegetables, fruit, beans, lentils, fish; moderate amounts of dairy produce, pulses and whole grains, and limited portions of red meat. A small amount of red wine has been shown to increase the health benefits. Keep sugar, soft drinks, confectionery, cakes, biscuits and puddings to a minimum. The pyramid illustration below is based on the dietary guidelines of Greece, which embrace the principles of the Mediterranean diet more closely than other countries.

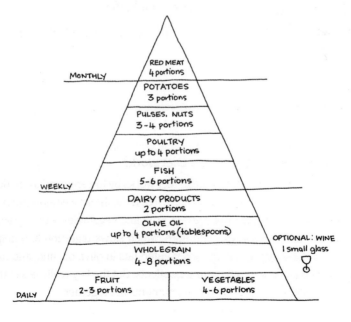

Daily

Olive oil: as the main added fat (up to 4 tablespoons)

Dairy: 2 portions (1 portion equals 150ml milk or yogurt; 25g cheese)

Fruit: 2–3 portions (1 portion equals 80–100g)

Vegetables: 4–6 portions (1 portion equals 80–100g)

Grains: (wholemeal bread, wholegrain pasta, rice etc.) 4–8 portions (1 portion equals 1 small slice of bread; or 25g uncooked pasta or rice)

Red wine (optional): 1 small glass (125ml)

Weekly

Potatoes: 3 portions (1 portion equals 100g)

Poultry: up to 4 portions (1 portion equals 60g cooked poultry)

Fish: 5–6 portions (1 portion equals 60g cooked fish)

Pulses, nuts, olives: 3–4 portions (1 portion equals 100g cooked pulses; 25g nuts)

Monthly

Red Meat: up to 4 portions (1 portions equals 60g cooked meat)

How to make the Mediterranean Diet work for you

You don't need to buy expensive out-of-season produce to gain the health benefits of the Mediterranean diet. Nor do you need to master Greek or Italian cookery. Mediterranean-style eating is more about the proportions of foods in your diet rather than eating particular foods. This means there is plenty of scope to be creative, using local and affordable produce, according to your taste. Just use the ingredient mix in any way you wish.

Focus on fruit and vegetables

Fruit and vegetables really are the mainstay of the Mediterranean diet. People in the Mediterranean average seven or more portions of fruit and vegetables a day, including at least one portion of green leafy vegetables such as spinach, rocket or watercress. They are normally cooked on the hob or roasted in olive oil, or eaten raw drizzled with olive oil. Studies found that older people who consumed a portion of cooked green leafy vegetables daily were half as likely to die in the next four years as those who ate no greens. In practice, this means having two or three vegetables with each meal.

Fruit and vegetables are high in fibre and bursting with vitamins, antioxidants and phytonutrients (plant nutrients that have beneficial health properties). Aim for at least seven portions a day by adding vegetables or salad to every main meal and fruit to breakfast and desserts. This is the amount associated with the longest lifespan. In a 2014 study of more than 65,000 people, those eating at least seven daily portions had a 42 per cent lower risk of death from any cause compared with people who ate less than one portion. And their risk of dying from cancer or heart disease was reduced by 25 per cent and 31 per cent respectively.

 DO IT NOW!

Adding fresh sliced berries, bananas, peaches or whatever is in season to your bowl of cereal or wholegrain cereal is an easy way to meet your seven-a-day target for fruit and veg. It not only adds sweet flavour, it also provides lots of satisfying fibre.

Antioxidants in fruit and vegetables help prevent or reduce cell damage caused by oxidation, a process that damages cells in the body and has been linked to the development of cancer, heart disease, Alzheimer's disease and Parkinson's disease. Several studies have linked a high intake of flavonoids – found mainly in fruit, vegetables and nuts – with a low rate of heart disease. Flavonoids are powerful antioxidants and have been shown to reduce the likelihood of blood clots forming.

A 2008 study by the Finnish National Public Health Institute showed that eating berries, rich in flavonoids, reduced platelet stickiness, increased HDL cholesterol and lowered blood pressure. Vitamin C-rich fruit also helps reduce furring of the arteries, according to a 2008 study by Norwegian researchers. Put this into practice with Blueberry Smoothie (page 153), Summer Fruit Compote with Yogurt (page 208) or Greek Salad Wraps (page 72).

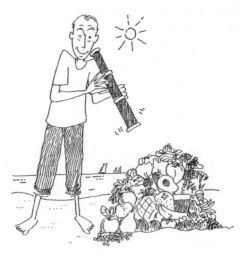

WHAT IS A PORTION? PART 1

✓ Fruit: 1 apple; 1 pear; 2 kiwi fruits; 1 tomato; 2 handfuls raspberries; 7 strawberries; 1 banana; 1 slice pineapple; 1 glass fruit juice; 1 orange; 1 nectarine; 2 satsumas; ½ avocado; 2 plums; 4 tablespoons blueberries

✓ Vegetables: 1 carrot; ½ pepper; ½ courgette; 1 cereal bowl raw spinach; 1 cereal bowl lettuce or salad leaves; 2 spears of broccoli; 2 handfuls cabbage; 3 tablespoons peas; 8 Brussels sprouts

(See also What is a portion? Part 2 on page 108)

The benefits of beans

Pulses (beans, lentils and chickpeas) often take the place of meat in many Mediterranean meals. They are high in protein, fibre, vitamins and minerals. Studies suggest that eating more pulses may help manage type 2 diabetes, prevent bowel cancer and reduce heart disease risk. A can of chickpeas can be whizzed up with a little lemon juice, olive oil and garlic to make houmous. Or you can add a tin of red kidney beans to a tomato and vegetable sauce, a tin of butter beans to a chicken and vegetable stew or a tin of lentils to a vegetable soup. Need more inspiration? Try Couscous, Chickpea and Goat's Cheese Salad (page 191), Lentil Chilli (page 200) or Fish with Spicy Chickpeas (page 183)

Go with the (whole)grain

Grains in the Mediterranean region are typically wholegrain and bread is an important part of the diet. However, throughout the Mediterranean region, bread is eaten plain or dipped in olive oil — not eaten with butter or margarine.

Make sure the grains you eat are mostly wholegrain varieties, such as oats, wholemeal bread, wholewheat pasta, brown rice, pot barley, quinoa (strictly a seed but nutritionally similar to grains) and bulgur wheat. As well as being rich in fibre, which helps to lower cholesterol and fill you up, they also contain lots of minerals such as iron. Refined ('white') grains, such as white flour, bread and rice contain less fibre, iron and B vitamins than whole grains (although, by law, white flour contains added calcium, iron and B vitamins to replace some of the nutrients removed during processing), which is why it's generally better to eat whole grain varieties. Their lower fibre content makes them less filling, so it's easy to overeat them. In a Harvard University study, women who ate at least two portions of wholegrains were 49 per cent less likely to be overweight than those who ate white versions. To get the most nutrients per portion, look for products that are 100 per cent wholegrain. Make breakfast healthier by swapping your usual cornflakes for Energy-Boosting Muesli (page 168) or Berry Porridge (page 166). Alternatively, swapping white pasta for the wholewheat kind – try Chicken and Vegetable

Pasta (page 176) or Pasta with Courgettes and Feta (page 193), or simply substituting plain white flour in recipes for wholewheat flour as in Healthy Banana Bread (page 207).

TO BE OR NOT TO BE... WHOLEGRAIN

It *is* a Wholegrain if it's called...	It's *not* a Wholegrain if it's called...
Wholegrain or brown rice	Cornflour
Buckwheat	Cornmeal
Bulgur or cracked wheat	Basmati rice
Millet	Enriched flour
Quinoa	Pumpernickel
Sorghum (cereal grain popular in Africa and Asia)	Long grain rice or short grain rice
Triticale (a hybrid of wheat and rye)	Rice flour
Wheat berries	Wheat starch
Whole-grain barley or pearl barley	Stone-ground wheat (if wholegrain, label should say 'stone-ground wholewheat')
Corn	
Oats or oatmeal	Unbleached wheat flour
Jumbo oats	Maize flour
Wholegrain rye flour	Wheat flour
Spelt	Corn flakes
Wholewheat	

Buying fruit and vegetables

With the Mediterranean diet the focus is on fresh, seasonal food that's affordable and locally produced. You don't need to spend a fortune on imported produce, much of which is harvested under-ripe before it has developed its full vitamin quota and may have lost much of its nutritional value during its journey to your supermarket. Include some seasonal British-grown fruit and vegetables, such as cabbage, cauliflower, apples and pears, in your diet too. They contain the same nutrients as Mediterranean produce, only in slightly different proportions. The key is to eat as wide variety as you can and make the most of produce that's in season. Here are some tips to keep in mind:

1. *Check fruit and vegetables are unblemished and undamaged* – these are signs that the produce hasn't been handled properly or that the food is past its best.
2. *Consider ripeness* – if you plan on eating the food later in the week, avoid buying produce that's too ripe. Similarly, make sure that the food you plan to eat today is ripe enough.
3. *Variety* – avoid getting into the rut of eating the same few fruits and vegetables. More variety means a better variety of nutrients. Bananas may be high in potassium but oranges and strawberries are high in vitamin C. You want to get them all.

 DID YOU KNOW?

Frozen fruits and vegetables are just as nutritious as fresh ones. They're usually picked ripe and immediately flash frozen, so they retain most of their nutrients. Stock up with frozen peas, spinach and green beans, as well as frozen berries (good for adding to smoothies or stirring in to porridge).

EAT A RAINBOW OF COLOURS

Vegetables	Nutritional benefits
Green leafy vegetables (e.g. rocket, cabbage, broccoli, cabbage, Brussels sprouts, kale)	High levels of vitamin C, potassium, fibre, calcium and carotenoids
Red, orange and yellow vegetables (e.g. peppers, butternut squash, carrots, pumpkin)	Contain vitamin C and carotenoids, important for healthy skin and for the immune system
White vegetables (e.g. onions, shallots)	Good sources of folic acid, fibre and potassium and flavanols that have anti-inflammatory and anti-cancer effects
Red and purple vegetables (e.g. aubergines, red cabbage)	Contain folic acid, fibre and anthocyanins, pigments that may help protect against heart disease

Fruit	Nutritional benefits
Red and yellow fruit (e.g. tomatoes, peaches, nectarines, plums, watermelon)	Rich in antioxidants and phytonutrients. Packed with vitamin C and lycopene, which may help reduce the risk of some cancers (lung, stomach and prostate)
White and green fruit (e.g. grapes, apples, pears)	Rich in potassium and soluble fibre
Orange fruit (e.g. oranges and satsumas)	Packed with vitamin C
Purple and red fruit (e.g. strawberries, blueberries, blackberries, raspberries)	Full of polyphenols, which help improve blood flow and have anti-inflammatory properties

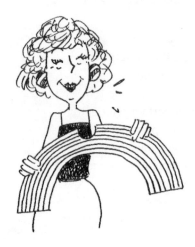

Swap your usual fats for olive oil

Olive oil is the main source of fat in the Mediterranean diet. According to figures from the International Olive Council, Greeks consume around 24 litres per person per year – Great Britain comes in at just over 1 litre.

Rich in monounsaturated fats – the type linked to improvements in HDL or 'good' cholesterol (which carries excess cholesterol from the arteries to the liver) – olive oil has anti-inflammatory compounds that contribute to healthy blood vessels. Studies have shown that olive oil can also help protect against osteoporosis – a disease that's uncommon in people in the Mediterranean who consume lots of olives and olive oil. One study in Spain also found an association between olive oil and protection against depression.

Make the swap by dipping your bread in olive oil (instead of spreading butter or margarine on it), and by drizzling it over salads and vegetables – use a teaspoon to drizzle on grilled or roast vegetables to boost the amount of fat-soluble nutrients you absorb.

Store in a cool dark place.

What are the different types of olive oil?
All olive oils contain the same calories and fat. However, virgin and extra virgin olive oils (the least processed forms) contain more polyphenols (antioxidants that may help prevent heart disease) and vitamin E.

Extra virgin olive oil (EVOO)
EVOO is the highest-quality olive oil and is made by cold pressing the olives. This means the oil is removed using only pressure and is not heated over a certain temperature. Cold pressing preserves the most flavour and polyphenols, and keeps the acidity under 1 per cent. EVOO has a low smoke point, which means it shouldn't be heated to high temperatures (and therefore not used for frying or roasting), but is perfect for drizzling on salads and finishing soups and pasta dishes.

Virgin olive oil
Virgin olive oil (without the 'extra') is produced through the same process but is made from slightly riper olives. It has a lighter flavour and is around 2 per cent acidity. Use virgin olive oil for cold dishes or low-temperature cooking.

Pure olive oil
Also labelled simply 'olive oil', pure olive oil is a mixture of refined olive oil and virgin olive oil. It still come from the 'first press' of olives but may be refined (heated) to remove undesirable odours and flavours and then blended with some virgin to be called 'olive oil' again.

Because of the heat used in the extraction process, this type of olive oil contains fewer antioxidants but still offers the same amount of monounsaturated fats as the rest of the oils. Use pure olive oil for everyday cooking, grilling, roasting and frying.

Light olive oil
Despite its name, light olive oil has just as many calories and just as much fat as the other types. The word 'light' refers to the fact that it's lighter in flavour — you don't get as much of that olive taste. This makes it a good choice for baking where you don't want an olive flavour. However, it can also be used for sautéing, grilling and frying. It has a high smoke point, which means it performs well at high temperatures.

CONVERTING BUTTER OR MARGARINE TO OLIVE OIL

To substitute olive oil for butter or margarine in cooking or baking, follow this handy conversion chart:

Butter or margarine	Olive oil
25g	20ml (1½ tablespoons)
50g	40ml (2½ tablespoons)
75g	60ml (4 tablespoons)
100g	80ml (5 tablespoons)
125g	100ml (6½ tablespoons)
150g	120ml (8 tablespoons)

WHY NOT TRY RAPESEED OIL?

Rapeseed oil is good in nutritional terms as a substitute for olive oil – it's produced in the UK, widely available in supermarkets and can be cheaper than some olive oils. Like olive oil, it is high in heart-healthy monounsaturated fats, but has considerably higher levels of vitamin E. It also boasts – at 6 per cent – a lower level of saturated fat than any other oil. It has a delicate, nutty flavour that keeps it versatile. It is delicious in dressings and dips, as well as in baking, frying and general cooking.

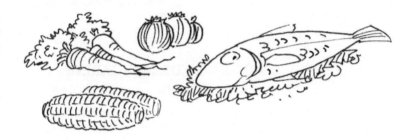

Eat fish at least twice a week

A key characteristic of the Mediterranean diet is fish. White fish is an excellent source of low fat protein while oily fish (such as salmon, mackerel and trout) contains omega-3 fats (see page 141). Omega-3s are vital for heart health – they reduce the stickiness of the blood, making it less likely to clot, and are linked to a lower risk of heart attacks. They also help to keep cell membranes healthy and have been linked to protection against depression. In areas of the world where people consume large amounts of fish, rates of depression are much lower than in regions where fish is rarely eaten. In a 2014 study, women who ate oily fish at least twice a week had a 25 per cent lower risk of having depression over a five-year period. For some tasty ideas, try Fish Minestrone (page 184) or Salmon with Roasted Mediterranean Vegetables (page 177).

TOP TIPS FOR BUYING, STORING AND COOKING FISH

Buying: Check that fish has bright eyes, a clean smell and that the flesh is firm, elastic and has a vibrant colour. The skin should look shiny and metallic and moisture on the fish should be clear, not milky. The fish may have been thrown around, so make sure all parts of it are intact. It should have a mild odour but not overpowering – don't buy fish that has a strong fishy smell.

Storing: Store fish in a sealed container on the lowest shelf of the fridge. This will stop it from touching or dripping on to other food and prevent the spread of harmful germs.

Cooking: Bake or steam fish rather than frying it, as the oils can become damaged at high temperatures. An easy method of cooking fish is to wrap it in foil or parchment (*en papillote*), throw in some sliced peppers, courgettes or mushrooms and a handful of fresh herbs, such as parsley or rosemary, put the package into a roasting dish and pop in the oven. It'll taste delicious and, what's more, there's no washing up. The important thing is to make sure you don't overcook fish. The white liquid that seeps out of the flesh is protein; if you see it then the fish is at risk of overcooking. If you're cooking the fish on the bone, use a little knife and pull it away from the bone – when it's cooked perfectly it'll come away easily.

Choose nuts for snacking

Regularly snacking on nuts in place of crisps or biscuits has been linked with numerous benefits including lower risk of heart disease, diabetes and even obesity. One study found a Mediterranean style diet supplemented with 30g nuts a day cut heart disease and stroke risk by up to half. Eating them even just once a week cut the risk by 7 per cent. Nuts contain healthy unsaturated fats, plant sterols and fibre – all of which help lower cholesterol levels.

Although nuts are calorific they are also satisfy hunger and can help control your appetite. One study showed that people who eat diets containing moderate amounts are more likely to maintain their healthy weight after dieting than those who don't. One handful of nuts (25g) a day will provide around 160 calories – choose plain or roasted nuts for healthy snacking (ideally, the unsalted kind). Add a handful of cashews to stir-fries (try Prawn and Vegetable Stir-Fry on page 185), some flaked almonds to your porridge (try Cinnamon Porridge with Banana and Nuts on page 167) or scatter a few pine nuts over your salad (try Couscous, Chickpea and Goat's Cheese Salad on page 191).

 DO IT NOW!

Nuts may be high in fat but that fat is the healthy monounsaturated kind, which has been shown to increase healthy HDL cholesterol levels and promote weight loss. According to one study, people who snacked on 42g nuts daily instead of a muffin with the same calories lost more weight from their midsections and had lower blood cholesterol levels after six weeks.

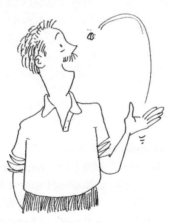

Enjoy a glass of vino

This is good news for those who enjoy alcohol in moderation although, of course, just because the Greeks and Italians drink wine it doesn't mean you have to take it up. The Mediterranean diet typically includes a moderate amount of wine; usually red wine, although white is also popular in some regions. Some of the heart benefits are due to a compound in the skin of red grapes called resveratrol, which is why red wine is thought to be better for the heart than white (see page 143). But, if you don't drink wine, then you can also get similar benefits from red grape juice and red grapes.

If you do drink it, try swapping your usual glass for a smaller one – that's a glass measuring 125ml for women, and 175ml for men. This may be somewhat less than you're used to – most bars and restaurants serve larger glasses nowadays and a 250ml glass is the norm in some places. And, let's face it, it's all too easy to pour much more generous measures at home. But it's worth checking your glass size and cutting back a little if necessary, as doctors say more than a small glass may increase the risk of health problems, including increased risk of certain types of cancer. As we get older, our 'resilience' to alcohol goes down and so we are more susceptible to its harmful effects. Here are some ways to reduce your risks:

- drink less than the upper limits advised by the NHS: three units a day and 14 units a week for women; four units a day and 21 units a week for men. A 125ml glass of wine contains 1½ units and a 175ml glass contains 2 units of alcohol
- avoid drinking at lunch if you are working in the afternoon
- have more days without than with alcohol
- have an occasional dry week, or do 'dry January'
- cut alcohol out or right down if you are trying to lose weight

Eat dairy foods in moderation
Although many Greeks start their day with yogurt and honey, the traditional Mediterranean diet contains far fewer dairy products than the typical British diet. People in the Mediterranean drink less milk than we do and eat only small amounts of cheese. Include about two portions of dairy products daily. One portion equals a small glass (150ml) of milk or a small pot of yogurt or a thin slice (25g) of cheese. If you're watching the calories, go for low fat products, such as skimmed or semi-skimmed milk and low fat yogurt. They

contain as much calcium as higher fat versions. Also, choose plain yogurt rather than sweetened flavoured yogurts. Make it tastier by scattering over some flaked almonds, or a handful of blueberries, some sliced bananas or a spoonful of raisins.

A 2014 study of more than 8000 people in the Mediterranean region found that those who consumed at least seven portions of yogurt a week were less likely to become overweight over a six-year period. This was even more pronounced in people who also ate a lot of fruit. These benefits are thought to be due to the calcium in yogurt, which helps prevent fat gain and speed up the weight loss process. Protein helps you feel fuller for longer and wards off hunger pangs. For an extra vitamin and fibre boost, do what the Greeks do – add a few chopped walnuts and a drizzle of honey.

Yogurt makes the perfect healthy snack or dessert. It provides calcium, protein and B vitamins. Just one small pot contains one third of your daily calcium needs, essential for strong bones. But some yogurts are high in fat and hidden sugars, so here's a guide to the credentials of the different types.

✓ Plain ('natural') yogurt: yogurt at its simplest, with no additional ingredients. The fat content can vary depending on the type of milk used, but low-fat plain yogurt has only around 2 per cent fat. Try adding extra fruit such as blueberries and a sprinkle of granola.

✓ Flavoured or fruit yogurt: this type of yogurt has 50 per cent more calories than plain and you get an average of two teaspoons of added sugar in each pot. But despite this, it raises blood sugar levels (due to its protein content) only very slowly which means it can curb hunger longer than sweets or biscuits.

✓ Light fruit yogurt: This yogurt is made with skimmed milk and sweeteners to achieve a lower calorie content but it's most likely to be loaded with additives.

✓ Live yogurts: most yogurts are 'live' or 'active' – in other words, they contain harmless live bacteria or active cultures – even if not stated on the label. These may help boost immunity and improve digestive health by boosting our good gut bacteria.

✓ Thick and creamy and custard-style yogurts are made with whole milk and cream and have a higher calorie and fat content than the low-fat type.

✓ Greek yogurt: Greek yogurt has a thick and creamy texture and contains around 10 per cent fat. If you're watching your weight, choose low fat (2–3 per cent fat) or fat-free varieties, or opt for *strained* Greek yogurt, which contains twice the protein of other yogurts (9–10 per cent as opposed to 4 per cent). Protein helps us to feel fuller for longer.

MEDITERRANEAN BREAKFASTS

To help your day get off to a healthy start here are four delicious breakfast alternatives to cereal:

1. Oats with Fruit and Nuts
   Combine 35g rolled oats with 100g low-fat plain Greek yogurt and leave overnight. Then stir in a handful of raspberries (or your favourite fruit).

2. Pomegranate and Berry Smoothie
   In a blender, whizz together a handful of berries, ½ banana, 50ml pomegranate juice and 125ml plain yogurt with a handful of crushed ice.

3. Greek Yogurt, Fruit and Honey
   Combine low-fat plain Greek yogurt with a tablespoon of chopped pistachios, some nectarine slices, a couple of chopped dried apricots and a drizzle of honey.

4. Scrambled Eggs Mediterranean-Style
   Beat 2 eggs with ¼ diced pepper, ½ tablespoon sun-dried tomatoes, ½ tablespoon sliced olives and 4 halved cherry tomatoes. Cook in a small non-stick pan over a moderate heat, stirring, until just set. Serve with a thin slice of wholemeal toast.

Eggs are eaten regularly in Mediterranean countries and are included in many cooked dishes. They are rich in high quality protein, vitamin D (for strong bones), selenium (cancer protective), zeaxanthin and lutein, both of which help prevent age-related loss of eyesight (macular degeneration). Eggs are one of the few sources of choline and B12, two nutrients that are important for your brain. Choline in particular has been linked with attention and memory. As one of the few natural sources of vitamin D, eggs are a good way to top up your intake without supplements (see page 151). See page 172 for our step-by-step guide to making perfect scrambled, poached and boiled eggs.

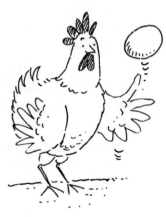

HOW MANY EGGS SHOULD YOU EAT?

The previous limits on egg consumption have been removed. For years we were warned about eating too many eggs due to their cholesterol content. But over thirty years of research has consistently found no relationship between dietary cholesterol or egg consumption and the risk of heart disease. Instead, we can blame high cholesterol levels on lifestyle factors such as excess weight, lack of physical activity and eating too many foods rich in saturated fats, all of which make our livers pump out too much LDL cholesterol. In fact, eating one or two eggs a day may even help with weight control, as eggs help increase satiety – the feeling of fullness after eating. Researchers found that people who ate eggs for breakfast went on to consume fewer calories at lunch and dinner than those who started their day with cereal or bagels. Over a longer period, this led to a greater rate of weight and fat loss.

Limit your intake of red meat

Red meat used to be a luxury item in rural parts of the Mediterranean, so people tend to eat it less frequently, perhaps as a side dish or as a way to flavour other dishes, hence its place at the very tip of the pyramid (see page 69). Limit beef, lamb and pork to no more than once a week if you can. Make sure it's not fatty by cutting off any excess fat before cooking, and keep portions small (about 60g, the size of a normal deck of playing cards). If you're used to eating mainly meat and two veg-style meals, then this may be a bit hard to start with. The easiest way to cut down is to swap meat for poultry or fish once a week, then twice a week. Try simple recipes like Salmon with Roasted Mediterranean Vegetables (page 177) or Easy Chicken Paella (page 181) to start with. If you're short on time then try something simple like Sardines on Toast (page 188) for example. Add pulses like beans and chickpeas to meals, such as Baked Sardines with Tomatoes and Chickpeas (page 180) or Mediterranean Fish Stew (page 182). You can also add red kidney beans, chickpeas and lentils to chilli, salad, soups and stews – you'll need less meat and your meal will still be filling and tasty.

 DID YOU KNOW?

Garlic is not only a great way of adding flavour to meals but it can also help improve blood circulation, improve cholesterol levels and lower blood pressure, all of which help cut the risk of heart disease and stroke. It may also boost your immunity and help combat flu and colds. These health benefits are thought to be due to the high levels of a compound called allicin, formed when a garlic clove is chopped or crushed – and which is responsible for the distinct smell. Be warned: if you are cooking garlic on the hob, do it slowly for a couple of minutes only. Don't burn it, as it'll turn bitter very quickly.

Why not try a 'meatless Monday' each week? – and see pages 189–200 for some vegetarian meal ideas – plant-based protein sources are often less expensive than meat, so it can be as good for your wallet as it is for your health.

IS RED MEAT GOOD OR BAD FOR YOUR HEALTH?

Several long-term studies have found that eating large amounts of protein from red meat and processed meat products may increase your risk of dying at an early age from heart disease, cancer or other diseases.

According to a 2012 study from Harvard School of Public Health, each additional daily portion of red meat (60g, about the size of a deck of cards) was associated with a 13 per cent higher risk of dying; each additional daily portion of processed meat products, such as salami, bacon, or hotdogs, increased the risk by

20 per cent. Researchers believe this could be due to red meat's saturated fat content as well as the salt and nitrates in processed meats. Nitrates are converted into nitrosamines in the body, which are carcinogenic.

Red meat has also been linked to an increased risk of bowel cancer. An analysis of 29 studies concluded that a high consumption of red meat increases risk by 28 per cent. This may be due to a lack of fibre among high meat consumers or to cancer-causing compounds called heterocyclic amines (HCAs) and polycyclic aromatic hydrocarbons (PAH) that form when meat is grilled, barbecued or roasted.

The NHS recommend eating no more than 70g of red meat (such as beef, pork and lamb) or processed meats (like ham, bacon and salami) per day.

Replacing the red meat you eat with delicious meals made with beans, lentils or chickpeas (try Chickpea and Butternut Squash Risotto on page 192 or Couscous, Chickpea and Goat's Cheese Salad on page 191) for just a few meals a week could have a really beneficial impact on your overall health.

The benefits of eating seasonally

People in the Mediterranean eat what they grow locally and therefore eat it when it's in season. Eating in-season food has many benefits. First off it's better for your body – foods picked and eaten when in season are higher in nutrients (especially vitamin C) than those flown in out of season from abroad. According to one study, spinach harvested in season contained around three times more vitamin C than out-of-season produce. Another found that the vitamin content of vegetables picked and frozen in season was significantly higher than fresh vegetables imported from Italy, Turkey, Spain and Israel.

Of course, you will also get more variety – you may eat a lot of one food while it's in season but when that season's over, you'll switch to other foods available at that time of year. Buying food available year-round in the supermarket means you can get stuck in a rut of eating the same kinds throughout the year, week in, week out.

It'll also give you a chance to explore some more creative cooking – having an abundance of one type of food, say spinach, means you'll have to find more ways of using it in your meals. This can make you more creative in your meal preparation.

Of course buying local gets you better value because you won't have to pay a premium for food that is scarce or has travelled a long way. Research has shown that a basket of fruit and vegetables bought in the summer can be as much as a third cheaper than the same basket bought out of season. It's also much better for the planet – seasonal produce has a lower environmental impact – growing fruit and vegetables in season requires lower levels of artificial inputs (heating, lighting, pesticides and fertilisers) than at other times of the year, and reduces the energy (and associated CO_2 emissions) needed to transport it across the globe.

What's in season when:

Vegetables

Spring: asparagus, carrots, celeriac, purple sprouting broccoli, savoy cabbage, spinach, spring greens

Summer: broad beans, beetroot, courgettes, fennel, green beans, peas, tomatoes, watercress

Autumn: mushrooms, marrow, pumpkin, squashes, sweetcorn

Winter: carrots, butternut squash, Brussels sprouts, cabbage, cauliflower, curly kale, leeks, swede

Fruit

Spring: rhubarb, gooseberries

Summer: blueberries, currants, plums, raspberries, strawberries

Autumn: apples, blackberries, pears, plums

Winter: apples, pears

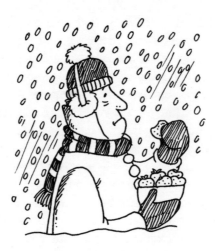

Summary of Eating the Mediterranean Way

- The traditional Mediterranean diet is regarded as the healthiest in the world.
- Eating the 'Med way' may help protect against chronic disease, cancer, type 2 diabetes, dementia and heart disease, as well as lead to a longer life.
- Eat more foods from plant sources: fruit, vegetables, unrefined whole grains, beans, lentils, nuts, seeds and potatoes.
- Keep sugar, soft drinks, confectionery, cakes, biscuits and puddings to a minimum.
- Focus on fresh and seasonal foods, ideally seven portions of fruit and vegetables a day.
- Eat more beans and lentils in place of some of the meat in your diet.
- Eat fish and poultry several times a week.
- Use olive oil to replace your usual oils and fats, such as margarine and butter.
- Limit red meat to no more than a few times a month.
- Eat dairy products and eggs in moderation.
- Enjoy a daily glass of wine (optional).

3

LOSE WEIGHT, GET IN SHAPE

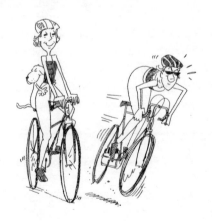

Carrying extra fat has a lot to answer for when it comes to shortening our lives and making us unwell. If you eat badly then you're storing up trouble. Being overweight or obese, particularly if you store excess weight around your middle, puts you at greater risk of developing:

- type 2 diabetes
- high blood pressure
- high blood cholesterol
- heart disease and stroke
- a number of cancers, including breast, womb, ovarian, bowel, kidney, colon and prostate cancer
- arthritis
- indigestion
- gallstones
- snoring and sleep apnoea

The good news is that losing weight, even a small amount, can help improve your health and lower your risk of developing these conditions. Whether you're trying to get back into your favourite jeans, planning to look your best for a family event, getting ready for a holiday or just fed up carrying around extra pounds, this chapter will help you reach your goal.

Maybe you've tried dieting in the past – and regained the weight you lost. Most people do – which just goes to show that diets don't work in the long term. That's because they usually focus on telling you what *not* to eat rather than what you *can* eat. And when you're told you can't eat something then – guess what? – you want to eat it more! So you give up the diet. The truth is, you don't have to drastically change your eating habits to change your weight. Studies show that making small tweaks rather than big ones is the key to keeping the pounds off. Swapping your daily glass of fruit juice for water, eating fruit instead of crisps and using smaller plates for your meals, for example, will save hundreds of calories a day and allow you to lose weight without making any big sacrifices. If you want to lose weight for good, then you have to make small changes to your diet, changes that can fit in with your lifestyle, changes that you can stick to.

 DO IT NOW!

Buy whole fruit rather than fruit juices. You'll feel fuller on fewer calories and get more healthy fibre from the actual fruit. A glass of apple juice, for example, has no fibre and more than 100 calories, but an apple has 50 calories and more than 3g of fibre.

This chapter will show you how to turn small lifestyle adjustments into major weight loss. It will give you lots of easy eating strategies and ideas for upping your activity levels, calorie-saving food swaps, meal ideas and simple tricks to avoid overeating and easy practical ways to exercise, so you can burn more calories. Before you know it you will have shed pounds and adopted healthy habits to last the rest of your life.

What is the difference between being overweight and obese?

You hear both the terms 'overweight' and 'obese' in the news a lot nowadays. Both refer to a condition of being over the weight considered healthy for your height and age. Being *overweight* means having more body weight than is considered normal or healthy. On the other hand, *obesity* means having an excess amount of body fat. Both conditions are measured by your Body Mass Index, or BMI (see below). People with a BMI of 25 or above are considered 'overweight'; those above 30 considered 'obese'. The numbers aren't an accurate measure of fatness, but rather a correlation between body fat, body mass and height.

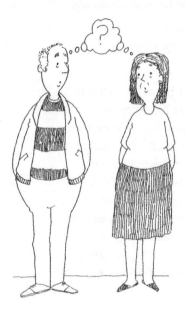

 DID YOU KNOW?

One in four people in the UK is obese and obesity rates have almost trebled in the last twenty years, according to Public Health England.

Do you need to lose weight?

You don't need to weigh yourself every day but you should use how you feel in your clothes and how you look in the mirror as an indicator of whether you need to lose some weight.

Alternatively, you can check your BMI. This measurement is used as an indicator of your health risks and is calculated by dividing your weight (kg) by the square of your height (m^2). For example, if your weight is 70kg and height 1.7m, your BMI is 24: $70 \div (1.7 \times 1.7) = 24$.

Alternatively, you can use the BMI calculator on the NHS website: www.nhs.uk/tools/pages/healthyweightcalculator.aspx

Your goal should be to maintain your BMI between 18.5 and 24.9.

- normal weight = 18.5–24.9
- overweight = 25–29.9
- obese = >30

People with a BMI between 18.5 and 24.9 have the lowest risk of developing diseases linked to obesity, such as heart disease, stroke and type 2 diabetes. The risk increases as your BMI gets higher. Although the BMI is effective indicator of how much fat you are carrying, it doesn't take into account *where* fat is stored in your body. This is important because 'apple' shaped people, who have most of their fat stored around the abdomen, are more at risk of developing obesity-related diseases than 'pear' shapes, who have most fat on their hips. The BMI also does not allow for how much muscle you have so is not an accurate method for assessing health risks for athletic people. Nor is it accurate for very slim or very overweight people.

 DO IT NOW!

Instead of eating chips... chop up some potatoes, put them on a non-stick baking tray, pour over a little olive oil and stick them in the oven at 200°C (180°C fan, gas mark 6) for 30 minutes. Hey presto, you will have delicious and much healthier wedges to eat.

What's the best way of calculating body fatness?

A better way of measuring your 'fatness' and risk to health is to measure your waist. Your waist measurement reflects the amount of fat you carry in your abdomen and is regarded as more accurate than BMI in predicting the risk of type 2 diabetes. Measure your waist midway between the top of your hipbone and the bottom of your ribs using a tape measure. This is not necessarily the same as your jeans or trouser size! Try the following tests to find out your health risk:

1. Waist measurement
As a rule of thumb, for women, if your waist measures more than 80cm (32in), and for men more than 94cm (37in), then you need to lose weight. Your risk of health problems is significantly higher if your waist size is more than 102cm (40in) (for men) or 88cm (34½in) (for women).

2. Waist to height ratio
Divide your waist measurement by your height. It should be no more than half your height. If your waist measures more than half your height then your health risks are higher and your life expectancy lower. For example, if you are 1.72m (5ft 8in/68in) tall, your waist size should be 86cm (34in) or less. If it's more than this then it's time to lose some weight.

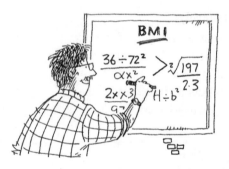

Why is fat around the waist a health risk?

A high waist measurement indicates excess visceral fat, the unseen fat in your abdominal cavity around your internal organs. The problem with this type of fat is that it doesn't just sit there. It actively alters the body's normal hormonal and chemical balances, pumping out hormones, insulin and inflammatory and clot-producing compounds. These changes increase levels of 'bad' LDL cholesterol, and also send signals that may cause cancer to grow. So a man with a 'beer belly' but slim limbs may be at greater risk of heart disease, type 2 diabetes and cancer than a pear-shaped person with the same BMI but less visceral fat.

DID YOU KNOW?

Obese women are nearly 13 times more likely to develop type 2 diabetes than women of normal weight; more than four times as likely to suffer high blood pressure; and three times as likely to develop cancer of the colon. Obese men are more than five times more likely to develop type 2 diabetes as those of normal weight; 2.6 times more likely to suffer high blood pressure; and about twice as likely to develop osteoarthritis.

Overweight and physical inactivity together account for about a third of all premature deaths, two thirds of deaths from cardiovascular disease and a fifth of deaths from cancer among non-smokers, according to a 2005 US study.

What causes obesity?

Scientists believe a number of factors working together cause obesity. Your genetic make up, pre-natal development, lifestyle and environment all have a role to play. But, whatever the contributory factors, you will deposit fat on your body if you eat more energy (calories) than you use. However, it is useful to consider the following factors.

1. Your predisposition

Researchers have found that genetics seems to play a part in regulating body weight. Many genes have been identified that either increase or decrease appetite as well as how fast or slow you burn the calories you eat. People who generally have little problem controlling their weight seem to have a precisely tuned appetite, while people who struggle to control their weight may be less sensitive to their body's signals of fullness. If you are overweight the chances are one or both of your parents were too. Children with two obese parents have a 70 per cent risk of becoming obese, compared with 20 per cent in children with two lean parents. This is partly due to genes but also the result of children taking on the same poor eating and activity habits as their parents.

Scientists believe that the nutritional signals you received before you were born affect your obesity risk in later life. Studies have shown that a high birth weight is a strong risk for becoming overweight. A 2005 US study found that children born to women who put on excess weight during pregnancy were more likely to become overweight themselves. Mothers who ate junk food during pregnancy and breastfeeding could also increase the child's chances of weight problems in later life, according to a 2007 UK study.

2. Your environment

The environment in which you live may not make it easy to make healthy lifestyle choices. The World Health Organisation uses a rather po-faced term for this, calling it an 'obesogenic environment'. Have you noticed how difficult it is to buy something healthy at service stations, for example? There's an abundant selection of chocolates and crisps but little in the way of healthy fruit and veg. The same goes for supermarkets, fast food restaurants, stations and cinemas, where tempting sweets, snacks and fizzy drinks are more prominently displayed than the fresh produce. Then there are the 'buy one get one free' special offers, enticing us to buy more biscuits – rather than nuts or bananas. Of course, no one's forcing us to buy these foods but the fact that they are available anywhere, anytime makes it harder to resist them. Thankfully, some supermarkets have replaced sweets at the checkout with healthier alternatives. Let's hope others will follow! Ever seen an advert on TV for potatoes or oranges? Probably not – companies don't make money from selling you simple vegetables and fruit but they do profit from potato crisps and orange juice drinks.

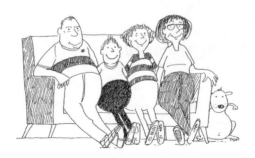

DO IT NOW!

In supermarkets, resist the temptation of buying jumbo packs and two-for-one offers of processed foods such as biscuits, desserts, ready meals, scones, cakes and crisps. You may tell yourself you'll only eat half the pack of crisps but the odds are you won't. Buy regular sizes or individually wrapped portions.

Another important factor concerning your environment is the drop off in activity as you get older. For most of us, physical activity is no longer a natural part of our daily lives. We're spending more time sitting at a computer or watching TV and we're generally far less active than we used to be. Did you know that the average person aged over sixty spends more than ten hours a day sitting? That not only means you're burning fewer calories but it also doubles your risk of developing type 2 diabetes and heart disease, according to a 2012 study of 800,000 people. Instead, you have to make time to exercise.

Think back to when you went to school – it's likely you walked or cycled or had to go by public transport, or regularly walked to the shops with your parents and spent your summer holidays playing outside. Maybe you keep to that same active lifestyle, but it's likely most of us spend more time in the car than we used to when we were younger (if our families even had a car when we were growing up!). According to a number of studies, people in the 1950s ate more calories than people today but were much slimmer because their daily lives involved far more physical activity. Most of our modern conveniences, such as cars, computers and home appliances, reduce our need to be physically active.

 DID YOU KNOW?

The average person burns around 300 calories an hour while going about their daily business. So, for example, if you walk for half an hour six days a week, you'll lose around a pound a month, without eating less – that's almost a stone a year.

3. Your decisions

Eating habits develop over many years, and are strongly influenced by our eating experiences in childhood. These are then continuously reinforced as we grow up, which makes them difficult to change. Were you always made to finish your plate even if you were full? Did you always have to eat pudding? Many of us grew up with a healthy diet of home-cooked food and meat and two veg but with increasing consumer choice, advertising and the advent of ready meals and shop-bought desserts, it became all too easy to overeat.

Overeating may be triggered by emotion. Some people turn to food in stressful situations such as after an argument or a difficult day at work. Have you ever noticed yourself venting your frustration on a bag of crisps or devouring a family sized bar of chocolate when you're upset? Other vulnerable times may be when you're bored or sad. Eating can also become a way of numbing the pain of unmet needs, such as love, comfort, security or control.

 DID YOU KNOW?

Having friends and family who are overweight raises your risk of being overweight too, according to a 2007 US study published in the *New England Journal of Medicine*. The data on more than 12,000 people over 32 years suggests the risk increases by 57 per cent if a friend is obese, by 40 per cent if a sibling is obese and 37 per cent if a spouse is obese. Of course, obesity isn't contagious in a physical sense, but having overweight family or friends changes your norms about what counts as an appropriate body size. It's easy to think that it is OK to be big when those around you are too.

How important is your metabolic rate?

Your *metabolic rate* is the rate at which your body burns calories. Your *basal metabolic rate* (BMR) is the rate at which you burn calories at rest on essential body functions, such as breathing and blood circulation. It accounts for 60–75 per cent of calories burned daily. The heavier you are, the higher your metabolic rate. BMR uses roughly 22 calories for every kilo of a woman's weight and 24 calories per kilo of a man's weight. Muscular people tend to have a higher BMR, as muscle burns more calories than fat. Genetics are also important – some people are born with a more 'revved up' metabolism than others.

Myths about Fatness

'Fat people have a slower metabolism than slim people'
In fact the opposite is true. The heavier you are, the higher your metabolic rate. It's a basic law of physics – larger people need more energy to pump the blood around the body and to keep moving. Just as bigger cars use more fuel than small cars, so bigger people use more energy than small people. The hard truth is slim people don't burn up calories any quicker – they just don't consume as many.

'Overweight people hardly eat a thing'
Many overweight people eat more than they think they do. A US study found that women typically reported eating 400 fewer calories than they actually consumed; one in four women under-reported by more than 800 calories. The more overweight the women the more calories they under-reported. Try measuring your food and keeping a food diary to see exactly what you eat and where your downfalls lie. Choose smaller portions of high calorie foods (desserts, biscuits, cakes) and fill up with foods that have a low calorie density (fruit, vegetables, salad).

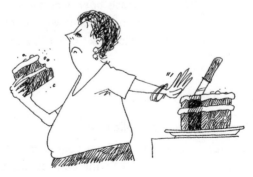

'Your genes make you fat'
Lots of people like to blame their genes when it comes to justifying their size. Indeed, fatness often appears to run families – if you're overweight then the chances are one or both of your parents are too. Scientists have identified a number of genes that favour a larger appetite or encourage fat storage. But genetic factors alone cannot explain the rapid rise in obesity rates. We all have the same genes we had twenty years ago, yet the number of obese people has doubled in this period. Clearly, it is changes in lifestyle and activity, rather than your genes that are responsible for making more people fat. Whatever your genetic make-up, you still have to eat more calories than you need to put on weight. The bottom line is that even if you are genetically programmed to gain weight more easily, you can still be slim. It's just that you may have to eat a little less than others or exercise a bit more.

LIFESTYLE VS. GENES

A number of populations in the world seem prone to obesity today. But they only become fat when their traditional lifestyle with its natural diet completely changed. For example, the Nauru Polynesians in the South Pacific rank as the fattest population in the world, with 1 in 3 suffering from diabetes. They became very obese when mining companies moved them off their home island. Their lifestyles became very sedentary and they began eating imported calorie-dense food. Their traditional diet of local fish, fruit and vegetables was replaced by a high fat Western diet of processed meat and refined carbohydrates and their genes made them especially vulnerable to obesity.

How can you lose weight?

We're not going to pretend that it's easy to change bad habits. But if you're going to change your diet it's best to make one or two small changes at a time. That way, you're more likely to stick with them in the long run. These changes should be things that you can comfortably live with, rather than quick fixes that you won't be able to maintain. Weight loss isn't about deprivation and you can still eat a little bit of what you fancy. Go slowly and follow these simple steps:

1. Set realistic goals

It's all very well saying you'd like to lose weight – you've probably said it to yourself a hundred times already – but unless you have definite goals then motivation is hard to find, and this is the key to success. Maybe set a weight-loss target for an upcoming event, such as a wedding or a birthday party, or something special like a holiday or a reunion to provide you with the necessary motivation. Setting a realistic goal will focus your mind and keep you on track. Without sensible goals, it's all too easy to slide back into those old habits.

Motivational tips:

- Write down your goal or tell someone else – such as a family member or a friend – what you want to achieve and why When it gets tough you can re-read these goals and it will keep you going.
- Believe in yourself – there is no reason you can't change, lose the weight you want to and feel happier.
- Plan your meals – it's vital that you get organised so that you have the right foods to hand and won't succumb to high-calorie snacks.
- Reward yourself when goals have been reached. Buying a new item of clothing or adding a tick to your food diary after reaching a weekly target will help you stay on track.
- Use family and friends – they can provide support and be a great source of motivation.

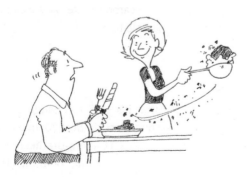

2. Start subtracting

The only way to lose body fat is to take in fewer calories than your body needs. As a rule of thumb, 3500 calories equals approximately 0.5kg (1lb) of body fat. That means you have to take in 3500 fewer calories than you usually do over a period of time to lose 0.5kg (1lb). Although this measurement is not 100 per cent accurate (your metabolism and therefore weight loss typically slows over time), it can serve as a useful guide if you are trying to lose weight.

By cutting your calories by 15 per cent, you'll lose fat not muscle. This should result in a healthy and steady weight loss. This means cutting about 300 calories if you normally consume 2000 calories a day. You can get an idea of how many calories you should be eating using the calculator on: www.healthstatus.com

Alternatively, you can estimate your daily calorie needs using the guide on page 14.

HOW MUCH WEIGHT CAN I LOSE A WEEK?

Experts agree that between 0.5 and 1kg (1–2lbs) per week is a healthy and effective rate of weight loss. A loss of more than 1kg (2lbs) per week means you could be losing muscle. *You should not cut your current calorie intake by more than 15 per cent.* A sudden drop in calories tells your body to conserve energy, as starvation might be imminent. Your body goes into survival mode and the rate at which you burn energy slows down. To compensate for the low calorie intake, your body will start to break down muscle tissue for fuel. So, you can end up losing muscle as well as fat.

3. Find out what you're *really* eating

Keeping a food diary for a few days will give you a much clearer idea of what you are really eating and where your calories are coming from. It's also a brilliant motivator – and means you cannot 'cheat'. Write down everything that you eat, noting the portion weights and sizes. Try to be as accurate as possible and remember to write down every snack and every drink. Be as honest as possible – that handful of crisps, those biscuits with your tea, that glass of wine with dinner. You may be surprised how many calories you eat or how often you nibble. Look at your food diary and identify the foods or drinks that really aren't helping your fat loss efforts. The main culprits are most likely to be high-calorie low-fibre snacks: biscuits, puddings, crisps, sweets, cakes and chocolate. Try to identify which foods you need to reduce or increase. Aim to eat as little sugar as possible and replace unhealthy snacks with fresh fruit and vegetables. This action will account for most of your calorie saving.

4. Eat more fibre-rich foods
To feel full on fewer calories, eat bigger portions of foods that are low in calories and naturally high in fibre – fruit, vegetables and salads. These foods make up a large part of the Mediterranean diet described in Chapter 2. They give maximum filling power for fewest calories, and thus help control your appetite and stave off hunger pangs. By increasing the amount of vegetables and fruit in a meal you can have satisfying portions for relatively few calories. Fibre expands in the gut, makes you feel full and helps stop you overeating. It also helps to satisfy your hunger by slowing down the rate that foods pass through your digestive system, which stabilises blood sugar levels. Studies have shown that people who increased their fibre intake for four months ate fewer calories and lost an average of 2.26kg (5lbs) – with minimal willpower. Try replacing half of your usual portion of potatoes or pasta with vegetables. That way you won't feel like you're eating less. Add extra vegetables to sauces, soups and stews as 'stealth' vegetables. Not only will they lower the calorie content of the portion you eat, they will also boost the nutritional content of the meal.

5. Eat less sugar
Avoiding sugary foods and drinks and reducing the amount of sugar you add to food and drinks will reduce the calories in your diet. The government recommends no more than 25g added sugars (6 teaspoons) a day (see page 25). Swap sugary desserts for fresh

fruit, swap sugar-rich drinks for water and calorie-free alternatives and check food labels for sugar – eat less of those containing more than 5g sugar per portion. The sugars found naturally in milk, yogurt and fruit do not count as added sugars. The best way to cut back on sugar is simply to avoid processed foods and satisfy your sweet tooth with fresh fruit instead. See page 29 for more sugar swaps.

TEN HEALTHY SNACKS

These tasty snack ideas will help keep hunger at bay. Better one of these than a packet of crisps or chocolate:

1. rice cakes with a little peanut butter

2. carrot, cucumber or celery sticks with salsa or houmous for dipping

3. a few almonds

4. plain popcorn

5. oatcakes with a thin slice of cheese

6. a handful of raspberries, blueberries or strawberries mixed with 2 tablespoons 0% fat Greek yogurt

7. fresh fruit

8. pre-made fruit salads – expensive but great to snack on when you're out and about

9. a banana

10. a couple of dried apple rings or figs and a few unsalted nuts

6. Eat (a little) more protein
Protein helps to make you feel fuller longer and so curbs your appetite (see page 33). Including a portion of protein-rich foods (such as meat, poultry, fish, eggs or beans) in each meal will help

satisfy your appetite while providing relatively few calories. The more satiated you feel after a meal the less food you will eat at the next one and the longer you will keep hunger at bay. Feeling full and satisfied while eating foods you like makes it much easier to lose those unwanted pounds.

 DO IT NOW!

Roasting a chicken? Rather than slathering it with butter before cooking, squeeze over some lemon juice and drizzle with 1 tablespoon of olive oil. And when the chicken's cooked, remember to remove the skin before eating, as most of the fat lies just beneath it.

Cutting back on fat in your gravy is also simple – just pour most of the fat out of the used roasting tin before you make gravy. Alternatively, invest in a gravy separator, which will split the fat from the meat juices so you can pour a sin-free version over your Sunday roast.

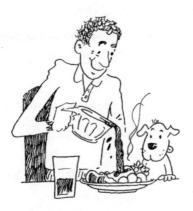

7. Think about portion sizes

Portion sizes have increased over the years, especially when it comes to ready meals, snack foods and restaurant meals. This means you may well be consuming extra calories without knowing it. It could be that you assume the portion given to you is the 'right' size. Or it could be that you are conditioned to finish everything that's on your plate. Perhaps you don't like to see food wasted or you were taught as a child to finish your plate. The problem is that you adapt quickly to eating bigger portions and don't tend to feel fuller as a result. Downsize fatty and sugary foods, and super-size fruit and vegetables.

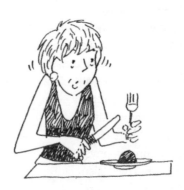

WHAT IS A PORTION? PART 2

Here is a guide to help you estimate portion sizes that fit in with the Mediterranean diet described in Chapter 2:

✓ one cupped hand = 1 portion (80–100g) of vegetables

✓ two cupped hands = 1 portion (80–100g) of salad

✓ size of a tennis ball = 1 portion (80–100g) of fruit, e.g. apple, peach

✓ one cupped hand = 1 portion (80–100g) of berries or chopped fruit

✓ size of a tennis ball = 1 portion of potatoes (100g)

✓ one small cupped hand = 1 portion (25g) nuts or seeds

✓ deck of cards = 1 portion (60g) cooked meat or fish

> ✓ size of 4 dice = 1 portion (25g) cheese
>
> ✓ one cupped hand = 1 portion (25g dry weight) pasta or rice
>
> ✓ 150 ml glass or cup = 1 portion of milk
>
> (See also What is a portion? Part 1 on page 72)

8. Step up your physical activity

The key to maintaining a healthy weight is combining healthy eating with exercise. Most of us can find the time to watch a film or go out for a drink, but finding the time to exercise seems so much harder. The simplest thing is to go for a walk a few times a week, starting off slowly and then building up your pace and distance. Try to build it into your daily routine, by walking short distances to the shops, for example, then gradually increase the time you spend walking.

Increasing the amount of physical activity you do will not only speed up weight loss but will also significantly lower your risk of heart disease, stroke, diabetes and cancer. Regular exercise helps reduce blood pressure and blood cholesterol levels, strengthens your muscles and bones, reduces stress and improves psychological well-being.

How much activity do you need to do for weight loss?

To keep your heart healthy and maintain fitness, experts recommend a minimum of 150 minutes (2½ hours) of moderate activity (such as walking or gardening) per week. This can be done as 30 minutes on at least five days a week. Or if this sounds too daunting, then divide your activity into shorter sessions – three 10-minute sessions of exercise produce the same fitness results as one 30-minute session.

However, for maximum health benefits and for weight loss, you should aim to do a bit more than this. To lose (rather than maintain) weight, the Department of Health recommends at least 60 minutes moderate activity most days of the week. A 2015 study published in the *British Journal of Sports Medicine* found that people aged over 65 who did three hours of exercise a week increased their life expectancy by five years compared to those who did less than one hour. And a 2015 analysis of studies involving more than 661,000 people found that those who did 450 minutes of light exercise (like walking) a week – or a little more than an hour a day – enjoyed the greatest longevity benefits. Better still, if you can include 20–30 minutes of more strenuous activity such as running or tennis, then you'll gain greater health benefits, according to a 2015 study by Australian researchers.

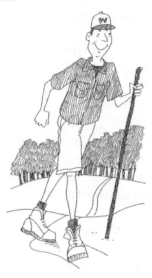

 DO IT NOW!

Try to spend an extra 30 minutes walking every day; this equals 4.5kg (10lb) weight loss a year:

☑ sitting burns 1 cal/min

☑ standing burns 2 cals/min

☑ walking burns 4 cals/min

Which type of exercise produces the fastest weight loss?

Aerobic, or cardiovascular, activities such as walking, running or swimming at an easy pace burn calories, but you will need to do them for quite long periods to burn enough to lose weight. Gradually stepping up the intensity will help you shed weight faster, as you'll be burning more calories per minute. In a study at the University of Wisconsin, women who cycled strenuously for 25 minutes each day lost the same amount of body fat as those who cycled at a more leisurely pace for 50 minutes each day.

If you are healthy and fit, then you may wish to try *high intensity interval training* (HIIT), alternating short bursts of intense activity (between 30 seconds and 2 minutes) with lower intensity intervals, during which you recover. This type of training has been shown to be most efficient for weight loss and building fitness. But this should only be attempted if you are already fit, otherwise you will risk injury. Even then, aim to do no more than one or two HIIT sessions a week, interspersed with moderate intensity sessions. Warm up at a low intensity then do one or two minutes of high-intensity alternating with two minutes of recovery. During your high intensity intervals you should be exercising hard enough to make carrying on a conversation difficult. Recovery intervals should be low enough to feel comfortable. As you progress, you can then start to increase the intensity or duration of the high intensity part and decrease the duration of the low intensity part. For example, if you're swimming, try alternating easy-paced lengths with some fast lengths. If you're walking, try speeding up or walking uphill for one or two minutes followed by one or two minutes of recovery – repeating this cycle three to times.

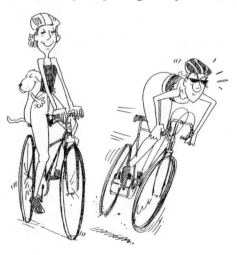

Before you start an exercise programme...

If you're over forty and recently inactive or have a heart condition or any health concerns you should consult a doctor before starting your exercise programme. If you're not sure where to begin, consult a qualified fitness professional who can advise on the right programme for you. See www.exerciseregister.org for a list of qualified exercise professionals.

EXERCISE PROGRAMMES AND WHAT THEY'RE GOOD FOR

If you have been less than active for the last few years of your life then it is essential to start slowly and build up. That way you will avoid injury and start to lose weight more effectively.

Good for...	Start with	Once you're fitter
... your heart	Walking, cycling, swimming, aqua aerobics	Aerobic and group exercise classes, running, tennis, hockey, circuit training
... your strength	Digging, swimming, hill walking, Pilates	Weight training, resistance bands, circuit training, body pump classes, Pilates, Ashtanga yoga
... keeping you supple	Stretch classes, beginner yoga classes	Yoga, t'ai chi, Pilates

Remember: Small Changes = Big Results

Downsize your dishes

Using smaller plates and bowls for everyday meals tricks your eye and brain into eating less. Using a larger plate or a larger serving spoon can cause you to dish up (and eat) larger portions. According to a Cornell University study, people given larger bowls served themselves 31 per cent more ice cream; when they used a large spoon they dished 15 per cent more into their bowls. And another study found that people who used short wide glasses poured 76 per cent more drink than when they used tall slender ones.

DO IT NOW!

While the oft-quoted small glass of wine at 85 calories doesn't sound too ruinous, in reality most bars and restaurants serve more generous-sized measures of 175ml (119 calories) and 250ml (170 calories). So, a couple of big glasses could cost you more than the calorie equivalent of a cheeseburger (299 calories).

Keep temptation out of the way

It may sound obvious, but if you want to avoid the temptation of high calorie snacks, don't buy them and don't have them in your house. Although you may think you can control your consumption, it's a lot easier if the only snacks in the kitchen are fruit and vegetables, rather than crisps and biscuits.

THINGS YOU CAN EAT (ALMOST) AS MUCH AS YOU WANT WITHOUT PILING ON THE POUNDS:

1. cantaloupe melon

2. strawberries

3. celery

4. cucumber

5. rocket leaves

6. miso soup

Slow down

Eating your food slowly and in a relaxed state of mind will curb your desire to eat more then you need. According to research at the

University of Florida, eating quickly means that the satiety centre in the brain doesn't receive the right signals and explains why you may feel hungrier sooner. Cut your food into smaller pieces, chew each mouthful thoroughly and don't load your fork with more food before swallowing the previous mouthful. Try putting down your knife and fork between mouthfuls.

Don't skip breakfast

People who skip breakfast thinking they're cutting calories are more likely to overeat later in the day and pile on unwanted pounds. Eating breakfast is a daily habit for the 'successful losers' signed up to the National Weight Control Registry. These people have maintained a 13.6kg (30lb) or more weight loss for at least a year, and some as long as six years.

Include protein, such as eggs, yogurt or milk, in your breakfast as this will help ward off hunger and keep you feeling full longer. If you want a bit of inspiration, see page 172 for a foolproof method for making perfect scrambled, poached and boiled eggs. One study published in the *International Journal of Obesity* found that people who ate eggs for breakfast for eight weeks (as part of a calorie-reduced diet) lost twice as much weight as those who started their day with bagels. The protein in eggs increases satiety and decreases hunger, which dramatically increases your chances of eating healthily throughout the day.

Here are some ideas for tasty high protein breakfasts of less than 300 calories:

- Bircher Muesli (page 169) or Energy-Boosting Muesli (page 168)
- Blueberry and Almond Yogurt (page 171)
- Berry Porridge (page 166) or Cinnamon Porridge with Bananas and Nuts (page 167)
- 150g low fat Greek yogurt with 25g nuts and a handful of blueberries
- 2 scrambled eggs on a slice of wholemeal toast
- 120g smoked haddock fillet with spinach and a poached egg
- 50g smoked salmon with 1 scrambled egg on a slice of wholemeal toast

Keep serving bowls off the table

To avoid overeating at mealtimes, serve your portion and then put any leftovers out of sight. Researchers found that when people are served individual plates of food as opposed to empty plates with a serving bowl in the middle of the table they eat 20–25 per cent less. If you don't have the dish on the table in front of you then there will be less temptation to keep refilling your plate. Get into the habit of freezing leftovers or putting them in the fridge immediately, away from temptation.

Don't be fooled by 'diet' or 'low fat' labels

If you eat food that looks like it should be high calorie or high fat but actually isn't, your body will soon cotton on. Experiments show that once it realises a food's appearance and taste promises don't match up to its calorie properties your body adjusts your hunger response so you no longer feel satisfied eating that food. The calorie savings of many low fat foods are small anyway, as sugar replaces most of the fat reduction. Studies show that people who consume large quantities of diet drinks have the highest intake of calories.

Eat without distractions

Rushing your food or eating in front of the television or computer screen almost certainly leads to overeating. When you're not concentrating on your meal it's harder to listen to your body and recognise when you are full. A 2013 review of 24 previous studies by British researchers concluded that eating while distracted could prompt you to eat more not only at that meal but later in the day, too. When people sat in front of a screen they consumed more snacks than those doing other things; they also consumed an extra 250 calories per meal more than those who ate without distractions. In a 2011 study people who ate lunch while playing a computer game consumed 123 more calories than those who did not. So always eat your meal at the table rather than having supper on the sofa. That way you can concentrate on the flavours and textures of the food and tune in to the signals your body gives you. After a few meals like this you'll soon have a good idea of when you've eaten enough.

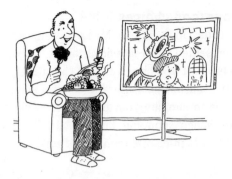

 DO IT NOW!

Eating meals in front of the TV causes people to consume about 250 calories more than those eating in quieter, less distracting environments, according to data published in 2013. So, eat your meals at the table.

Don't ban your favourite foods

Cutting out favourite treats, such as chocolate and cake, is more likely to make you put on weight than lose it, according to a survey. In fact, 86 per cent of slimmers lost weight while continuing to enjoy their favourite treats. The moment you tell yourself you can't have something – whether it's chocolate, crisps, cake – you want more of it. Even if you eat other things, you'll still want that forbidden treat and eventually you'll give in and have it anyway. If you know that you can eat a little of your favourite indulgence every day, you'll stop thinking of it as a forbidden food and then won't want to binge on it.

 DO IT NOW!

Have fewer takeaways. But if you must, then have a ready meal and boil or steam lots of vegetables to eat with it.

Simplify your food choices

Research at Tufts University in Massachusetts shows that when people are presented with a wider variety of foods they eat considerably more. If you have lots of different foods on your plate you prolong the sensory pleasure, which stops you feeling full. The message here is to simplify your diet. Place fewer types of foods on your plate. When shopping, stick to your list and ignore the temptation of any high-calorie foods that catch your eye.

 DO IT NOW!

Try fat-free flavourings – squeeze orange or lemon juice into stews or over meats; add citrus zest, soy sauce, fresh ginger, chilli peppers, herbs, or tomato sauce to your favourite recipes.

Thirsty or hungry?

That afternoon stomach pang or feeling of fatigue may be your body's way of asking for a glass of water, not a bag of crisps. How can you tell? When you feel the urge to eat, try drinking a glass of water (or another no-calorie drink) and see how you feel 10 minutes later.

Fill up with soup

Starting your meal with a bowl of soup can cut your calories by 20 per cent compared with eating the main course alone, according to Pennsylvania State University studies. It doesn't matter whether you choose a chunky or a smooth/puréed soup; but it should be a low calorie variety providing no more than 150 calories per portion (such as vegetable soup, which was tested in the studies) rather than a creamy one. The fibre and liquid fills your stomach, so you then go on to eat less food.

Start meals with salad or fruit

Eating salad or fresh fruit as a starter can cut the number of calories you eat in your main meal by 12 per cent, according to a 2004 study at Pennsylvania State University. All that fibre and water takes the edge off your appetite, so you eat less of the higher calorie foods in the main meal. The reason is that we tend to eat a fixed weight of food every day, regardless of calorie or nutrient content.

Ditch the juice

Eat the whole fruit instead and opt for water, sugar-free drinks or tea instead. Fruit juice contains much higher concentrations of (natural) sugar than the fresh fruit it comes from, and is less satiating. When you squeeze the fruit you lose the filling power of fibre. Even crushing it to make a smoothie destroys the cell walls, so you don't have to chew the fruit. This means it's easy to over-consume calories before your hunger is satisfied. Drinking a glass of orange juice gives you about 120 calories, but if you eat an orange instead you'll save 60 calories, get more fibre and feel more satisfied.

Take a walk before dinner

Taking gentle exercise, such as a walk, before a meal is not only a good way to burn a few calories but it can also help you eat less. In a study of overweight women conducted at the University of Glasgow, 20 minutes of walking reduced appetite and increased sensations of fullness as effectively as a light meal.

Go with the (whole)grain (again)

The fibre present in the wholegrain content of brown bread, pasta and rice prolongs the digestion process so sugar is released over a longer period of time. According to a Harvard University study of 74,000 women, those who ate more than two daily servings of wholegrains were 49 per cent less likely to be overweight than those who ate white versions.

Drink water before a meal

Drinking water before a meal reduces feelings of hunger so you automatically eat less. In one study, older adults who drank two cups of water before a meal lost roughly 2kg (4lb) more than those who didn't. Yet another study found that women who increased their water consumption while they dieted lost more weight than those who drank less than one litre a day. The European Food Safety Authority recommends 1.5 litres of water for men and 1 litres of water for women per day, but this can come from food (like fruit and veg), plain water and other drinks.

THE GOOD GUYS

Here are five foods that reduce your appetite naturally:

1. Avocados
   Rich in vitamin E and monounsaturated fats, avocados can actually help you eat less – the fats in these fruits send signals to your brain that tell your stomach that it's full.

2. Almonds
   A rich source of antioxidants, vitamin E and magnesium, a 43g daily serving of almonds has been shown to decrease hunger and help people maintain their weight loss, according to a 2013 study at Purdue University in the US.

3. Apples
   Their high content of soluble fibre and pectin help you feel full, as well as regulating your blood glucose level. They also require lots of chewing time, which helps slow down your eating and give your body more time to realise you're no longer hungry.

4. Eggs
   Studies have shown that eating an egg or two for breakfast can help people feel fuller than if they eat a bowl of cereal or a croissant with the same calories. Those who ate eggs ate 315 fewer calories over the course of a day than the cereal-eaters.

5. Milk
   Rich in whey protein, which is one of the most satiating nutrients. One study found that people consume fewer calories at their next meal after a milk-based drink.

Calorie Swaps

By making a few easy swaps in your diet you can save calories and drop pounds. As a general rule, cut down on sugary, processed foods, such as cakes, biscuits, pastries, chocolates, sweets and puddings, and sugary drinks. These foods are loaded with calories and are easy to over-consume because they don't really fill you up.

Instead, choose unprocessed foods rich in nutrients and naturally filling: fruit, vegetables, salad, milk and dairy products, fish, lean meat, poultry and wholegrains. Keep a check on portion sizes, especially when eating out, and always include the calories in drinks in your daily tally. Here are ten easy swaps to get you going.

Swap ...	For this	And save ...
1 slice (100g) cheesecake	125g plain yogurt with 100g fruit	300 calories
1 slice apple pie	110g stewed apple	110 calories
1 bag crisps (30g)	30g plain popcorn	100 calories
1 rasher streaky bacon	1 rasher trimmed back bacon	40 calories
1 slice (75g) chocolate cake	1 apple	295 calories
1 Mars bar	1 banana	180 calories
Chicken korma (350g)	Chicken tikka (350g)	230 calories
2 digestive biscuits	2 satsumas	96 calories
200ml apple juice	Water	76 calories
330ml cola	Water	135 calories

SWAP ICE CREAM FOR YOGURT

In one study from the University of Tennessee, dieters who ate three servings of yogurt a day lost 22 per cent more weight – including 81 per cent more fat in the stomach area – in 12 weeks than those who did not. They also retained one-third more lean muscle mass, which can help you maintain weight loss.

Now keep it off!

Now that you've lost the weight, you need to build a few good habits to avoid piling the weight back on. Here are six strategies used by the 10,000 people on the US National Weight Control Registry who have successfully lost at least 13.6kg (30lb) and kept the weight off for at least a year:

1. Eat 50 to 300 calories less than most people each day.
2. Exercise (gently) for an hour or more a day – the equivalent of a 4-mile walk.
3. Weigh yourself regularly and cut back if your weight goes up more than 1kg (2lb).
4. Eat breakfast every day and don't skip meals – doing this will stop hunger pangs and over-eating.
5. Spend no more than 10 hours a week watching TV.
6. Be consistent – don't 'cheat' on weekends or holidays.

BE SHOP SMART

✓ never shop when hungry – you'll be more likely to fill your trolley with snacks and unhealthy food

✓ change your route around the supermarket – spend more time around the perimeter where the fresh foods are usually found, and less in the centre where there's all the processed packaged foods

✓ plan for the week and try to stick to a shopping list

✓ try shopping online, it's easier to avoid temptation

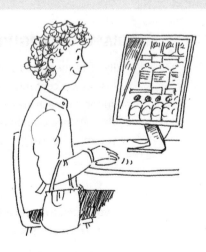

Summary of Lose Weight, Get in Shape

- Are you overweight? If your waist is more than 94cm (37in) for men or 80cm (32in) for women then you probably need to lose weight.
- Carrying too much fat around your middle puts you at greatest risk of heart disease, type 2 diabetes and cancer.
- Set yourself realistic weekly or monthly goals. Motivation is the key to success.
- The only way to lose body fat is to take in fewer calories than your body needs. Eat about 15 per cent less and aim to lose between 0.5 and 1kg (1–2lbs) per week.
- Keeping a food diary is a good motivator.
- Eat more foods that are low in calories and naturally high in fibre – fruit, vegetables and salads.
- Cut right down on sugar, especially sweetened drinks; avoid processed foods and satisfy your sweet tooth with fresh fruit instead.
- Include some protein-rich foods (such as meat, poultry, fish, eggs or beans) in each meal to help curb hunger and make you feel fuller, for longer.
- Downsize fatty and sugary foods, and super-size fruit and vegetables.
- Move more – the simplest thing is to go for a walk a few times a week. Aim for 30 minutes a day five times a week. Adding high-intensity intervals will produce greater fitness gains.
- Small changes add up to big ones. These include not eating in front of the TV, using a smaller plate, slowing down your eating, never skipping breakfast, eating salad before your main course and swapping biscuits for fruit.

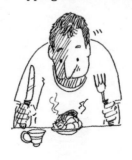

4

EAT YOURSELF WELL

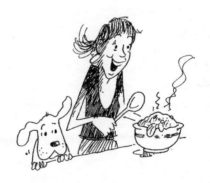

It's all too true that you are what you eat, and the food you consume can either make you healthy or unwell. We've seen the effects that our diet can have on the way we feel, from combating stress and tiredness to boosting energy levels and immunity. But when it comes to dodging major diseases the evidence is stronger than ever that our food can play a major role. The food we eat is the cause, wholly or partly, of many of our modern epidemics, such as heart disease, type 2 diabetes and some cancers, including bowel cancer. Many of these conditions are preventable. By eating a healthy diet, exercising more, and not smoking or drinking too much, you can dramatically reduce your risk of developing them. Eating the right kinds and combination of foods gives you a much better chance of staying healthy well into old age.

The World Health Organisation's Global Strategy on Diet, Physical Activity and Health estimates that a staggering 80 per cent of cases of heart disease, 90 per cent of type 2 diabetes cases and one third of cancers can avoided by changing to a healthier diet, increasing physical activity and stopping smoking.

This is good news – changing the way you eat can have a big impact on your health. Take charge in the kitchen – banish the sugary snacks and processed foods, and reintroduce some healthier options into your shopping trolley. Learn in this chapter about some easy switches and changes you can make to improve your diet and reap the rewards!

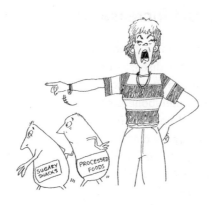

Reducing your risk of disease

While there are certain risk factors that you have no control over, such as your predisposition to illness and your family history of disease, there are still many ways of reducing your risk of chronic diseases. These centre around your eating habits, how active you are, how much exercise you take, whether or not you smoke and how much alcohol you consume. Perhaps one of the biggest things you can do to cut your risk of disease is maintaining your weight within a healthy range. Being overweight puts strain on your organs, including your heart, liver and digestive organs and greatly increases your chance of developing high blood pressure, high blood cholesterol and type 2 diabetes – all of which make it more likely that you will develop cardiovascular disease (such as heart disease and stroke), certain cancers and joint problems. In short, being overweight sends you down a rabbit hole of health problems. If you are already at a healthy weight, aim to keep it that way by eating a healthy diet and taking regular exercise. Being as little as 5kg (11lb) over your ideal weight range can significantly increase your risk of the diseases mentioned, no matter how slim you were in your younger years. To know whether or not you need to lose weight, look in the mirror and be honest! Or go by the feel of your clothes. Does the waistband on your trousers feel tighter than it used to? If the answer is yes, then you need to start making a few changes to what you're eating – see Chapter 3 for some simple tips.

Conditions that increase risk

The following conditions are not so much diseases in their own right as risk factors for disease. These are features of a condition called the metabolic syndrome, which, as explained in the book *Sod Seventy!* is the main metabolic problem that affects people in their sixties, seventies and beyond. It refers to a combination of being overweight, having type 2 diabetes, high blood pressure and raised levels of cholesterol. It puts you at greater risk of heart disease, stroke and other conditions affecting blood vessels. On their own, these conditions may simply harm your blood vessels, but having all of them together (which is quite common) is particularly dangerous. About one in four people are estimated to have metabolic syndrome. It is mainly the result of years of consuming too many calories and not taking enough exercise. The good news is that there is plenty you can do to prevent or even reverse these conditions.

High Blood Cholesterol

A high level of cholesterol in the bloodstream increases the risk of heart disease and artery disease. According to the NHS a high level of total blood cholesterol is judged to be above 5.0mmol/l (millimoles per litre). But knowing your cholesterol level isn't enough to tell you your personal risk of heart disease. Usually, when you have your blood cholesterol measured, your GP will look at your total cholesterol level, plus your LDL and HDL cholesterol. These are special molecules that transport cholesterol around the body. And it's the balance of these lipoproteins, rather than your overall total cholesterol level, that matters.

What the difference between LDL and HDL cholesterol?

Around 70 per cent of the cholesterol in your blood is carried on *low-density lipoproteins* (LDL). These carry cholesterol from the liver to the body cells, where the cells take as much cholesterol as they need, leaving any excess in the blood. If there's constantly too much LDL left in the blood it can build up in the arteries, eventually causing blockages or breaking away to form clots – this is why it's often referred to as 'bad' cholesterol. A high level of LDL cholesterol is defined by the NHS as above 3.0mmol/l. As a rule, the higher your LDL cholesterol level the greater the risk to your health.

The remaining cholesterol in your blood is carried on *high-density lipoproteins* (HDL). This is the 'good' stuff, as it picks up and removes excess cholesterol back to the liver for elimination from the body. High levels of HDL are associated with a *low* heart disease and stroke risk. The greatest danger is when someone has high levels of LDL cholesterol, and low levels of HDL cholesterol. Your ratio of total cholesterol to HDL may also be calculated. This is your total cholesterol level divided by your HDL level. Generally, this ratio should be below four, as a higher ratio increases your risk of heart disease.

Healthy levels of cholesterol are:

- Total cholesterol – below 5mmol/l
- LDL cholesterol – below 3mmol/l
- HDL cholesterol – above 1mmol/l

How can I lower my LDL cholesterol level?

Keeping a healthy stable weight, taking enough exercise, eating a healthy diet and not smoking will all help lower your cholesterol levels. Cutting down on saturated fats and trans fats, and replacing them with monounsaturated fats and omega-3 fats, both of which lower LDL levels, will also help. Eating more soluble fibre (found in oats, beans, lentils, fruit and vegetables), which lowers cholesterol by binding with fat and cholesterol in the gut and stopping it being absorbed, as well as eating more fruit and vegetables rich in antioxidants, which help prevent LDL being deposited on blood vessel walls, are other options.

Canadian researchers found that when people with high cholesterol levels consumed at least four daily portions of foods containing soluble fibre (such as oats), soy, almonds and plant sterols (natural compounds in grains, vegetables, fruit, nuts and pulses that can lower blood cholesterol) their cholesterol levels dropped by an average 14 per cent after 12 weeks. They also suggested that regularly eating cholesterol-lowering foods could cut cholesterol levels by more than 20 per cent, results similar to those seen with statins (cholesterol-lowering drugs).

THE GOOD GUYS

Here are four of the best cholesterol-lowering foods:

1. Soya foods
   Soya foods such as soya beans, soya milk alternative, tofu and edamame beans (unripened green soya beans) contain

soluble fibre as well as compounds called isoflavones, which have a positive impact on cholesterol levels. These are natural compounds that mimic the effects of oestrogen in the body and as a result will raise HDL levels. Studies have shown that including at least 15g of soya in your daily diet reduces blood cholesterol by 6 per cent. You can get this amount from two 250ml glasses of soya milk or 75g tofu.

2. Oats and barley
Oats and barley are rich in a type of soluble fibre called beta-glucan. This forms a gel that binds cholesterol in the intestines and prevents it being absorbed, thus helping lower levels of cholesterol in the blood and reducing the risk of heart disease. Soluble fibre also helps slow the digestion and absorption of carbohydrates, reducing blood sugar and insulin levels. High levels of blood insulin are associated with a higher heart disease risk. It is recommended that we eat about 3g of beta-glucan per day to lower blood cholesterol. You can get this from 90g oats, 6 tablespoons of oat bran or 9 oatcakes. For a healthy start to the day, try Overnight Oats (page 170) or Energy-Boosting Muesli (page 168).

3. Nuts
Nuts are rich in protein, fibre, heart healthy unsaturated fats, vitamin E, magnesium, potassium, natural plant sterols and a host of beneficial plant nutrients. Eating 30g a day – about a handful – can lower cholesterol by an average of 5 per cent. This is equivalent to about 25 almonds, 25 cashews or 30 peanuts. Add a handful of almonds to your porridge, a handful of cashew nuts to stir-fries or stir roasted peanuts into a curry.

4. Plant sterols and stanols
Plant sterols and stanols have a similar structure to cholesterol. They occur naturally in many vegetable oils,

including soya, rapeseed, corn and sunflower oil as well as nuts and seeds. They are also added to spreads, yogurt drinks, milks and yogurts. Popular brand names include Benecol and Flora Proactive. Plant sterols work by blocking the absorption of cholesterol from the intestines, thus reducing LDL cholesterol levels in the bloodstream. You can expect a cholesterol reduction of around 10 per cent in 2–3 weeks if you consume between 1.5–2.4g per day. Less than this amount probably won't provide much benefit, according to a 2004 study at Washington University. There's no additional benefit in taking more than 3g a day. You can get 2g from a 67.5g shot of sterol-fortified yogurt drink, a 125ml pot of sterol-fortified yogurt, two 250ml glasses of sterol-fortified milk or two servings of sterol-fortified spread.

Should I cut out foods containing cholesterol?

For most people, there is no need to limit cholesterol-containing foods such as liver, kidneys, eggs and prawns. New research has found that cholesterol in food actually has very little effect on blood cholesterol levels. Since the liver makes most of the body's cholesterol, when you consume cholesterol, the liver simply makes less. On the other hand, when you consume saturated fat, the liver makes more LDL cholesterol and so blood cholesterol levels rise. According to Heart UK, *cutting saturated fat rather than cholesterol* is a better way to keep your blood cholesterol levels within healthy limits. Only people who have an inherited condition called familial hypercholesterolaemia, where the body cannot regulate its cholesterol production so effectively, should avoid cholesterol-rich foods.

So remember – reduce your consumption of saturated fat, and up your consumption of cholesterol-lowering foods – like oats, nuts, fruit, beans and lentils. Try Berry Porridge (page 166) or Overnight Oats (page 170) for breakfast, a handful of nuts to snack on and a Benecol yogurt after a meal!

High blood pressure

High blood pressure – or hypertension – means that your blood pressure is consistently higher than the recommended level. Over time if it is not treated it increases your chances of having a stroke or heart attack. One in three people have high blood pressure and each day 350 people have a preventable stroke or heart attack caused by the condition. Having high blood pressure means your heart has to work harder to push the blood around your body. And this extra pressure puts extra strain on your arteries, which can weaken. Not doing enough physical activity, being overweight, consuming too much salt, drinking too much alcohol and having a family history of high blood pressure can all increase your risk of high blood pressure.

What do the numbers mean?

Your blood pressure is measured in millimetres of mercury (mmHg) and consists of two figures. The top number – *Systolic blood pressure* – is the pressure of the blood on your artery walls when your heart contracts and pumps blood through your arteries. The lower number – *Diastolic pressure* – is the pressure of the blood on your artery walls when the heart relaxes between beats.

High blood pressure is usually defined as having a systolic pressure of 140mmHg or more and a diastolic pressure of 90mmHg or more. A blood pressure reading below 130/80mmHg is considered to be normal.

How can I lower my blood pressure?

You can lower your blood pressure by making a few simple changes to your diet as well as being a healthy weight, taking regular exercise, not smoking and sticking to safe alcohol limits. Both the Mediterranean diet and something called the DASH (Dietary Approaches to Stop Hypertension) diet plan, developed by US researchers, have been proven to lower blood pressure. The DASH diet is similar to the Mediterranean diet – both emphasise fruit, vegetables, fish, nuts, seeds, whole grains, beans, lentils and olive oil – though the former includes a larger amount of lean meat and low fat dairy products. By closely following the Mediterranean or DASH diets, you may be able to reduce your blood pressure by a few points in just two weeks. Over time, your systolic blood pressure could drop by 7–12 points, which can make a significant difference in your health risks. Here are three features recommended in both diets that will help lower your blood pressure:

Cut salt

The quickest ways to lower your blood pressure are by cutting down on salt and losing weight. Eating too much salt makes your body retain water, which can raise your blood pressure. As we get older our bodies can't regulate fluid levels so well and our sensitivity to salt increases. This means excess salt may cause an above-normal rise in blood pressure. Three-quarters of the salt in the average diet comes from processed foods such as bacon, ham, sausages, sauces, ready meals and crisps. See page 53 for the salt content of popular foods. Check the labels of food for salt and aim to consume no more than 6g daily (see page 57). A high salt food carries a red colour code on the front-of-pack label, and contains more than 1.5g per 100g. Be aware that many foods that don't taste salty, such as breakfast cereals, cakes and biscuits, can still contain high levels of salt.

 DO IT NOW!

If you are in your sixties or seventies and have high blood pressure, it is essential that you cut down the amount of salt you are used to using. Here are some simple tips to get control of salt consumption:

☑ avoid foods containing more than 1.5 g salt per 100g – these carry a red colour code on the front of the pack

☑ wean yourself off adding salt to cooking or at the table – hide the salt cellar!

☑ use herbs and spices such as garlic, oregano and lemon juice to add flavour to meals instead of salt

☑ avoid cured and smoked foods such as bacon, ham and smoked haddock

☑ limit salty processed foods such as ready meals, ready-bought sandwiches, burgers, sausages, pizza, takeaways, sauces and savoury packet snacks like crisps and tortilla chips

Eat more fruit and vegetables

By eating more fruit and vegetables, you will increase your potassium levels and help to balance out the negative effects of salt. This will help your kidneys to work more efficiently – and help to lower your blood pressure to a healthy level. In a 2014 study of 90,000 post-menopausal women, those with the highest potassium intakes were 12 per cent less likely to suffer a stroke than those consuming the least. The World Health Organisation recommends a daily intake of 3510mg potassium, which you can obtain from five portions (400g) of fruit and vegetables a day (see page 46). It is best to get your daily potassium from natural sources, such as fruit and vegetables rather than taking supplements.

Drink alcohol in moderation

Staying within the NHS recommended levels for alcohol will help reduce your blood pressure. The NHS recommends men should not regularly drink more than three to four units a day and women should not regularly drink more than two to three units a day. Alcohol is also high in calories, which can make you gain weight and, in turn, increase your blood pressure.

THE GOOD GUYS

Research has found that drinking 250ml of beetroot juice daily can reduce blood pressure. The high content of nitrates in beetroot produce a gas called nitric oxide in the blood, which widens blood vessels and results in a modest reduction in blood pressure. You can find beetroot juice in most supermarkets or reap similar benefits from the whole vegetable – roasted, steamed, in soup or grated raw in salads.

Other lifestyle changes that will help to lower your blood pressure

- Don't smoke – smoking is the single biggest avoidable cause of high blood pressure, heart disease and stroke. If you need help giving up try your local NHS stop smoking services (www.nhs.uk/smokefree) or the NHS Smoking Helpline (available on 0300 123 1044).
- Get more exercise – the British Heart Foundation recommends doing at least 30 minutes of moderate activity at least five times a week. This can be broken into segments of 10 minutes each. See *Sod Sixty!* and *Sod Seventy!* for more ideas on how to get active.
- Reduce stress levels – blood pressure can increase with stress.
- Have your blood pressure checked regularly – there are usually no symptoms associated with high blood pressure so it is possible to have it for a long time and not know about it.

Type 2 diabetes

Over 3 million people in the UK have been diagnosed with type 2 diabetes and more than half a million have it but have not been diagnosed. It is a condition where the body cannot control the amount of glucose in the blood because of problems with the hormone insulin. When blood sugar levels are raised, there's an increased risk of glucose attaching to and damaging tissues. Diabetes is a serious condition, which, if left untreated, can lead to complications such as heart disease, blindness, kidney failure and nerve damage in the legs. Not many people realise that having diabetes can reduce your life expectancy by up to 10 years. Fortunately, if you spot the symptoms early you can reduce your chances of serious problems.

Type 2 diabetes can be managed with lifestyle changes such as a healthier diet, weight loss and regular physical activity. Insulin tablets and/or injections may also be required to achieve normal blood glucose levels in some people. Making some simple changes to your diet will help to improve your health and protect against long-term damage to the eyes, kidneys, nerves, heart and major arteries.

WHAT'S THE DIFFERENCE BETWEEN TYPE 1 AND TYPE 2 DIABETES?

Type 1 diabetes develops if the body is unable to produce any insulin. It is treated with regular insulin injections as well as a healthy diet and regular physical activity. It usually affects people under forty years of age. Type 2 diabetes develops when the body can still make some insulin, but not enough, or when the insulin that is produced does not work properly (known as insulin resistance). It is usually associated with being overweight and is found mostly in adults – although in recent years more children are being diagnosed with the condition. It can be managed with diet and physical activity, although some people may also need tablets or injections.

How do I know whether I am at risk of diabetes?
More than 80 per cent of people with type 2 diabetes are overweight. The more overweight and the more inactive you are, the greater your risk. Excess fat around your waist also puts you at high risk. For women, if your waist measures more than 80cm (32in), for men, if your waist is more than 94cm (37in) then you are an increased risk of diabetes. Other risk factors include:

- type 2 diabetes in your family
- high blood pressure, or having had a heart attack or stroke
- polycystic ovary syndrome

- being overweight
- impaired glucose tolerance or impaired fasting glycaemia (high levels of blood sugar, see page 24)
- a history of gestational (pregnancy) diabetes (a type of diabetes that some women get during pregnancy)

Do people with type 2 diabetes need to follow a special diet?

You do not need to eat special foods or meals. Essentially, you should eat plenty of high fibre foods, such as vegetables and fruit; and limit your intakes of processed foods high in sugar and fat, such as biscuits, cakes and crisps. Fibre is really helpful – it can slow the rate at which carbohydrate in foods enter the bloodstream and so improves blood glucose control. In fact, eating our favourite – the Mediterranean-style diet (see Chapter 2) – can lower your risk of developing diabetes in the first place by 83 per cent, according to a 2008 Spanish study. If you are diagnosed the aim of your diet needs to be to control blood glucose levels, achieve normal blood lipid (fat) levels, maintain a healthy blood pressure, maintain a healthy weight and prevent or slow the development of diabetes complications.

I've been diagnosed – what can I eat?

The single most important step you can take is not being overweight, or to lose weight if you are. Here are some general eating rules for preventing and managing type 2 diabetes but, if you have been diagnosed with the condition, you should seek advice from a registered dietitian with expertise in diabetes care:

- Eat regular meals throughout the day – avoid skipping meals – this will help you maintain blood sugar levels within a healthy range. If you are the kind of person who skipps breakfast – don't! You need to eat a combination of carbohydrate, protein and fats, such as Overnight Oats (page 170), Bircher Muesli, (page 169) or Cinnamon Porridge with Banana and Nuts, (page 167) to prevent blood sugar lows that lead to hypoglycaemia

- Include at least five portions of fruit and vegetables in your daily diet, including green leafy vegetables, which have been shown to be protective against type 2 diabetes (due to their high levels of polyphenols and vitamin C, both of which have antioxidant properties)
- Contrary to popular belief, there's no need to cut out carbohydrates completely. Adjust serving sizes according to the recommendations of your doctor or registered dietitian. If you're active then you'll need to eat more than someone who isn't
- Include beans, lentils and oats in your meals – these foods help maintain blood sugar levels within healthy limits. Try Energy-Boosting Muesli (page 168), Berry Porridge (page 166), Fish with Spicy Chickpeas (page 183) or Chickpea and Butternut Squash Risotto (page 192)
- Swap some saturated fat for unsaturated fats such as olive or rapeseed oil, oily fish, avocado, seeds and nuts
- Keep added sugars to a minimum (see page 23) – but you don't have to cut it out completely; any sugar you do eat should be eaten in nutritious foods such as yogurt and fruit rather than sweets or cakes
- Avoid sugary drinks – sugar in drinks is the most harmful form of sugar as it is rapidly absorbed and can cause a spike in blood sugar, which can make you gain weight in the long term. Instead drink water or sugar-free drinks
- Eat at least two servings of fish a week, including at least one meal of oily fish such as salmon, mackerel or sardines
- Eat less than 6g salt a day by cutting down on processed foods (see page 131)
- Limit alcohol to 21 units weekly for men and 14 units weekly for women. Have at least two alcohol-free days per week

AS A DIABETIC, SHOULD I CARRY DEXTROSE TABLETS AROUND?

Only people on insulin need to carry and use sugary snacks when they are going hypo (suffering from hypoglycaemia or low blood sugar). Generally, people with type 2 diabetes will not go hypo and do not need to take such precautions.

Does sugar cause diabetes?

Eating sugar does not directly cause diabetes. Diabetes is caused by a combination of genetic and lifestyle factors. Research concludes that the issue is eating too many calories – including those from sugar – that can lead to weight gain, which greatly increases the risk of type 2 diabetes. Studies show that drinking sugary drinks is linked to type 2 diabetes. Adding one extra serving of a sugary drink a day increases your risk by 26 per cent, according to a 2015 European study. So avoid squash, fizzy drinks, fruit drinks, energy drinks and sports drinks as far as possible.

Diet related Diseases

The same risk factor can cause more than one disease and one disease may be caused by more than one risk factor. Here is what you can do to reduce your risk or to prevent further decline in function due to cardiovascular disease, cancer and osteoporosis.

Cardiovascular Disease

This is an umbrella term for heart disease, stroke, angina, heart failure, cardiomyopathy and atrial fibrillation. Heart disease is the main cause of death in the UK – nearly one in six men and one in ten women die from it each year – that's 200 people each day or one every seven minutes. Stroke is also a major killer – it causes more than 40,000 deaths each year and 1.3 million people in the UK have had a stroke. Smoking, being overweight, having a high level of cholesterol in your blood, high blood pressure, diabetes, stress and being physically inactive increase your chances of developing heart disease or stroke. Eating better may reduce your chances of developing heart disease and stroke by:

- keeping your weight in the healthy range
- lowering your blood pressure
- lowering levels of LDL cholesterol
- increasing levels of HDL cholesterol
- preventing blood clots that can lead to heart attack and stroke

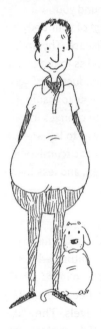

Five key healthy eating rules for cutting your risk of heart disease and stroke

1. Maintain a healthy weight

Maintaining a healthy and stable weight is one of the most important ways of reducing your risk of heart disease and stroke. Being overweight puts strain on your organs, including your heart. It is estimated that overweight and physical inactivity together account for two thirds of deaths from cardiovascular disease. Having a Body Mass Index (BMI) greater than 25 (see page 95) greatly increases your chances of developing type 2 diabetes, high blood cholesterol and high blood pressure – all of which make it more likely that you will develop heart disease or stroke. If you are already at a healthy weight, aim to keep it that way.

I HAVE A BIT OF A PAUNCH BUT MY LEGS AND ARMS ARE SLIM – IS THIS A PROBLEM?

Having excess fat around your waist ('apple-shaped' obesity), whether or not the rest of your body is slim, is considered a big risk factor for heart disease. The problem with this type of fat is that it has easier access to the blood supply of the liver. It increases the liver's production of very low-density lipoproteins and reduces its sensitivity to insulin (which increases the risk of type 2 diabetes). These changes increase the risk of heart disease and stroke. A simple way to tell whether you are 'apple-shaped' is to measure your waist circumference. It should be less than 80cm (32in) for women, and less than 94cm (37in) for men.

2. Swap some saturated fat for unsaturated fat
Swapping some of the saturated fat in your diet for unsaturated fats – found in nuts, seeds, olives (and their oils), avocados and fish – can protect your heart because these healthy fats raise HDL and lower LDL cholesterol levels. They also improve the ratio of total cholesterol to 'good' HDL cholesterol, lowering the risk of heart disease. A 2012 review of studies from the Cochrane Collaboration found that people who did this for at least two years reduced their risk of heart attacks, angina and stroke by 14 per cent.

As a general rule, it's a good idea to keep your intake of saturated fats low. The Department of Health recommends getting less than 10 per cent of calories from saturated fat. This means trimming the fat from meat, eating less processed meat (such as sausages, bacon and salami), and cutting out fatty processed foods (such as biscuits, cakes, pastries and pies). But you don't have to eliminate saturated fats from your diet completely. New research suggests that those found in dairy products, butter and eggs are not as harmful. While they raise LDL, they also raise 'good' HDL cholesterol so the overall effect on the heart is neutral.

But don't overdo it and start *adding* butter to your diet. Butter is still high in calories so keep portions small. Olive and rapeseed oils are healthier options than butter as they lower LDL and raise HDL cholesterol; and low-fat milk and yogurt are good choices (if you're watching your weight) because they have fewer calories and just as much calcium as full-fat versions.

Avoid anything that has 'hydrogenated oils' in the ingredients list, this is simply a code name for trans fats.

IS A LOW FAT DIET THE HEALTHIEST DIET FOR MY HEART?

Despite popular belief, a low fat diet is not the healthiest one for your heart. Instead a *moderate* fat diet containing mostly unsaturated fats is now thought to be more protective. A 2006 study involving 49,000 people published in the *Journal of the American Medical Association* found no difference in heart disease between people eating a low fat diet and those who didn't. Scientists now believe that it is the *type* of fat we eat not just the *amount* that's important when it comes to the risk of heart disease. People who eat a moderate fat diet containing nuts and olive oil have been found to have healthier blood cholesterol levels than those following a low fat regime. So remember, it's all about eating the RIGHT fat – fat (of the right kind) is NO LONGER A DIRTY WORD.

3. Eat a Mediterranean diet

We keep coming back to this. Study after study has shown that people who follow a traditional Mediterranean diet have a lower rate of heart disease and stroke, and live longer. In general, they consume less saturated fat (such as butter, meat and cheese) and more monounsaturated fats (such as olive oil, nuts and avocados), which is more beneficial than a diet that's low in fat. They eat lots of fruit and vegetables, oily fish, low amounts of red meat and dairy foods, plenty of whole grains, beans, nuts and seeds, olive oil as a source of fat and drink only small amounts of wine (see Chapter 2).

A 2015 study by Greek researchers found that that people who adhered strictly to a Mediterranean diet were 47 per cent less likely to develop heart disease over 10 years than those who didn't. A 2013 study in Spain found that people following a Mediterranean diet had a 30 per cent lower risk of heart disease and stroke and suggested that it was *almost as good at reducing the risk of a heart attack as taking statins*. Another study, the Lyon Diet Heart Study published in 2001, looked at the diets of 600 heart attack survivors. After four years, those following a Mediterranean-style diet had a 50–70 per cent lower risk of recurrent heart disease. The health benefits are thought to be due to the unique combination of foods in the diet rather than to single nutrients.

CAN OMEGA-3S CUT MY HEART ATTACK RISK?

There is plenty of evidence to suggest that people with the highest intakes of omega-3s have the lowest risk of heart disease and stroke. Omega-3s can help reduce the stickiness of the blood, making it less likely to clot. They also help the blood flow more easily through the smallest blood vessels, reduce blood fat (triglycerides) levels and help raise HDL cholesterol levels, which protect against heart attacks. You should aim to eat oily fish, such as sardines, mackerel, salmon, fresh (not tinned) tuna, trout and herring at least once a week. Alternatively, you can get your omega-3 quota from a tablespoon of walnuts or pumpkin seeds, one teaspoon of flaxseed oil, one tablespoon rapeseed oil or two omega-3 eggs (from hens fed an omega-3 enriched diet) a day.

4. Eat plenty of fruit and vegetables
Fruit and vegetables – a key feature of the Mediterranean diet – are packed with antioxidants, which help protect against heart

disease. These include beta-carotene, vitamin C, flavonoids as well as hundreds of other nutrients. Antioxidants mop up free radicals (see page 69), which can cause furring of the arteries. Both WHO and UK dietary guidelines recommend eating five portions of fruit and vegetables a day to help cut the risk of heart disease.

Several studies have linked a high intake of flavonoids – found mainly in fruit, vegetables and nuts – with a low rate of heart disease. Flavonoids are powerful antioxidants and have also been shown to reduce the likelihood of clots forming. A 2008 study by the Finnish National Public Health Institute showed that eating berries, rich in flavonoids, reduced platelet stickiness, increased HDL cholesterol and lower blood pressure. Vitamin C-rich fruit also helps reduce furring of the arteries, according to a 2008 study by Norwegian researchers. So, instead of eating biscuits or crisps, you should snack on berries and nuts to boost your antioxidant intake.

FOLIC ACID AND HEART DISEASE

Much recent research on heart disease has focused on folic acid. That's because it has been shown to reduce blood levels of homocysteine, an amino acid that is a natural by-product of the breakdown of protein. Raised homocysteine levels in the blood damage the cells that line the arteries, increasing heart disease risk. The good news is that upping your intake of folate – a B vitamin found in green leafy vegetables (such as spinach, cabbage and rocket), whole grains, beans, lentils and liver – reduces the risk. So try adding a handful of spinach to a hearty stew, a chicken curry or a simple risotto. Swap lettuce for a handful of rocket in sandwiches and wraps. For inspiration, try One-Pan Spanish Fish Stew (page 187) or Goat's Cheese and Beetroot Salad (page 197).

5. Stick to healthy alcohol limits
Its all too easy to consume more alcohol then you realise, especially when pouring your own drinks at home when there's no measuring

guide (and no one looking) – one glass of wine or whisky can be 3–4 units of alcohol. The NHS advises a maximum of 3 units a day and 14 units a week for women; and a maximum of 4 units a day and 21 units a week for men (see page 149). Drinking more than these levels increases health risks. While a little alcohol (just one or two units a day – the equivalent of a small glass of wine or half a pint of lager or beer) may give some protection against heart disease, this is due in part to its ability to increase levels of 'good' HDL cholesterol and reduce platelet stickiness, but any more increases your risk of heart disease.

Wine is favoured in the Mediterranean diet for its heart-health benefits. Both white and red contain compounds that have powerful antioxidant effects but red wine appears the most protective due to its high content of polyphenols, saponins and a compound called resveratrol. These compounds may help lower LDL cholesterol and stop blood platelets from clumping together, thus affording greater heart disease protection. All red varieties contain these beneficial compounds but pinot noir grapes – grown in the Chilean valleys, Bordeaux and Burgundy in France – have especially high levels of resveratrol.

Some good news for the over sixties – research has found that these benefits are limited to men over sixty and post-menopausal women. They do not apply to younger people – alcohol may severely impair their physical and mental development. Women are more vulnerable to the effects of alcohol than men. Because they have more fat and less water in their bodies, alcohol is absorbed more quickly and they are more susceptible to its toxic effects.

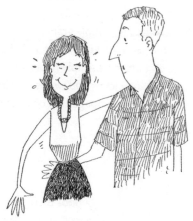

IS TOO MUCH MEAT BAD FOR YOUR HEART?

Red meat and processed meat are major sources of saturated fat in the average person's diet, and have been linked to an increase risk of heart disease. For example, in 2012 researchers from Harvard School of Public Health in the US found that people who eat red or processed meat regularly are more likely to develop conditions leading to heart disease. Each daily serving of red meat (a serving is judged to be roughly about the size of a deck of playing cards) increased the risk of heart disease by 18 per cent. A 2013 study of half a million people across Europe found that people who ate more than 160g of processed meat a day – roughly two sausages and a slice of bacon – were 44 per cent more likely to die over a 12-year time period than those who ate less than 20g. But you don't have to cut out red meat completely – stick to the UK government recommendations of no more than 70g of red meat (such as beef, pork and lamb) or processed meats (like ham, bacon and salami) per day. Try swapping red meat for a chicken fillet or piece of fish, or swapping ham in your sandwich for tuna or cheese. And lots of people are trying to have at least one meat-free evening meal a week – go to page 190 for some delicious vegetarian suggestions.

Cancer

Around one in three people in the UK develop cancer at some point during their lifetime. But there is a huge amount of research that shows you can reduce your cancer risk by changing what you eat, being more active and maintaining a healthy weight. The largest review of links between diet and cancer, incorporating the findings of 7000 research studies from all over the world, was published by the World Cancer Research Fund (WCRF) in 2007. It concluded that there is convincing evidence that diet plays a role in many cancers. According to Cancer Research UK, one in ten cancer cases could be prevented by eating more healthily.

Seven ways to cut your cancer risk

Experts say that by following the recommendations of the WCRF report you could reduce your risk of cancer by about a third. These recommendations include:

1. Stay a healthy weight

Maintaining a healthy weight is the most important step you can take to reduce your cancer risk. A healthy weight is defined as having a Body Mass Index (BMI) below 25 (see page 95). A healthy waist measurement is less than 80cm (32in) for women and less than 94cm (37in) for men.

The WCRF advises being at the lower end of the normal BMI range (between 21 and 23), or 'as lean as possible without becoming underweight'. This might sound difficult but it is what the science is saying more clearly than ever. Putting on weight can increase your cancer risk.

Being even slightly overweight increases your risk of a range of common cancers including bowel, breast, oesophagus, pancreatic and kidney cancer. According to a 2015 statement from the American Society of Clinical Oncology, one in five cancer deaths are caused by obesity. Cancer Research UK found that breast cancer risk could be as much as double in post-menopausal women who are overweight. This is because fat cells release hormones such as oestrogen, which increase the risk of breast cancer. But fat stored around the waist is the most risky because it encourages the body to produce 'growth hormones' that makes cancer cells grow. If you need to lose weight, see pages 91–122 and remember the key rules – eat less and exercise more.

2. Avoid high calorie foods and sugary drinks

The WCRF recommends cutting down on calorie-dense foods that are high in fat and sugar, such as chocolate, crisps, chips and biscuits. The main problem with these foods is they are easy to over-consume, increasing the risk of weight gain and obesity, which in turn increases the chances of developing a range of cancers including bowel and breast cancer. A 2003 Canadian study involving 580,000 women found that eating lots of fatty foods, particularly those high in saturated fat, increases the risk of breast cancer by 20 per cent.

But the WCRF report warns against sugary drinks in particular. The problem with sugary drinks is that they don't make you feel full, so you keep eating and drinking, even though you've consumed enough to keep you going for a while. A 2013 study found that the more sugary drinks a woman drinks the greater her risk of contracting endometrial cancer. Those who drank more than four servings a week (and that includes fruit drinks and fruit juices) had a 78 per cent greater risk of developing cancer than those who drank none.

Instead of sugary drinks and fruit juice, try water with a slice of lemon, orange or lime. Or opt for sparkling water – it's sugar-free, calorie-free and just as hydrating (it's a myth that it erodes tooth enamel or saps calcium from the bones).

WILL EATING SUGAR MAKE CANCER WORSE?

No, it's a myth that people with cancer shouldn't eat sugar because it causes cancer to grow faster. According to the National Cancer Institute, sugar doesn't speed the growth of cancer nor does depriving cancer cells of sugar slow their growth. However, a high-sugar diet may contribute to weight gain and obesity may increase the risk of developing several types of cancer.

3. Put plant foods first

Base your diet on plant foods, such as fruit, vegetables, whole grains and pulses. These foods protect against a wide range of cancers including mouth, stomach, lung, prostate and pancreatic cancer. As well as containing vitamins and minerals, which strengthen the immune system, plant foods are also good sources of phytonutrients. These are natural compounds that help to protect body cells from damage that can lead to cancer. According to Cancer Research UK, one in twenty cancers in the UK are linked to diets low in fruit and vegetables.

According to the WCRF report foods rich in fibre decrease the risk of bowel cancer. It recommends eating wholegrains or pulses (beans and lentils) with every meal. The European Prospective Investigation into Cancer and Nutrition (EPIC) study by Cancer Research UK and the Medical Research Council involving more than half a million people in ten European countries found a clear link between the amount of fibre eaten and the incidence of bowel cancer – those with the least fibre in their diets had the biggest risk. A 2007 study at the University of Leeds found that women eating 30g fibre a day halved their risk of breast cancer compared with low fibre eaters (less than 20g).

But certain vegetables are particularly protective against cancer. These include broccoli, cabbage and cauliflower, which contain indole-3-carbinol and genistein. These compounds boost the body's ability to repair damaged DNA and may prevent cells turning cancerous, according to a 2006 study from Georgetown University in the US.

So try to make vegetables, beans and lentils the centre of your meal – and remember that broccoli, cabbage and cauliflower are superfoods! See page 196 for a great meal idea.

MORE MEDITERRANEAN MAGIC

At the risk of sounding like a broken record, adopting a Mediterranean diet may cut your cancer risk. Researchers have found that people living in countries such as Spain and Greece where they generally eat more vegetables and fish, less red meat and cook in olive oil, have lower rates of cancer. A 2008 study of 26,000 Greek people found that eating less meat and more pulses cut the risk of cancer by 12 per cent. Using more olive oil alone cut the risk by 9 per cent. And a 2015 study of 5000 women found that those who stuck closely to the Mediterranean diet had a 57 per cent lower risk of endometrial cancer. Beans, lentils and nuts are a key feature of the diet, both of which are rich in a compound, inositol pentakisphosphate, which has been shown to inhibit the growth of tumours.

FOOD AND CANCER

What to avoid	What to eat
Ham, bacon, pastrami, salami, hot dogs, sausages – all strongly linked to bowel cancer	Broccoli and Brussels sprouts – contain sulphoraphane, which protects against cancer
Fast foods, biscuits, cakes – high fat and sugar foods are linked with obesity and several cancers	Carrots, tomatoes, mangoes – contain beta-carotene, which helps the immune system fight cancer
Smoked, cured and barbecued food – linked to stomach and oesophagus cancer	Beans, lentils, wholemeal bread, brown rice and wholemeal pasta – for fibre, aim to get three portions a day
Fizzy drinks, squash, cordial – the WCRF warn against all sugary drinks	Sardines, mackerel, herring, salmon – good substitutes for meat; contain omega-3 fats which fight cancer
	Brazil nuts – contain cancer-fighting selenium
	Soya milk/yogurt – a rich source of phytoestrogens, which may block the cancer-causing effects of your own oestrogen

4. Don't eat much meat

The WCRF considers processed meat and red meat the biggest culprits when it comes to bowel cancer risk. The big Europe-wide EPIC study found that the more meat people ate, the greater the risk of bowel cancer. Bowel cancer was 30 per cent more common among people who ate two daily 80g servings of red and processed meat, compared with those who ate less than 20g. And French researchers found that every daily 80g serving of processed meat increased bowel cancer risk by two-thirds. Something called 'haem' compounds found in red meat trigger the formation of carcinogenic (cancer-causing) N-nitroso compounds in the gut. About 500g (5 palm-sized portions) of red meat (beef, lamb and pork) a week is fine but more than that might increase your risk of bowel cancer, according to the WCRF.

The WCRF report states that eating just 50g a day of processed meat, such as sausages, bacon and ham, increases your cancer risk by 21 per cent. They recommend cutting out all processed meats. The problem is the nitrates in the meats, which lead to the formation of carcinogens in your bowel. But salt, which is often added to processed meats, may also play a role. It may promote inflammation in the stomach, which can lead to cancer. Cured and smoked meats also contain carcinogenic substances that can damage body cells and lead to cancer.

Replace some of the meat in your diet with other protein sources, such as beans, chickpeas and lentils. Make them the centrepiece of your meal – try making Chickpea and Butternut Squash Risotto (page 192) or Couscous, Chickpea and Goat's Cheese Salad (page 191). They will make you feel full and you shouldn't miss the meat element of the meal. You could also try adding them to curries, salads, casseroles, chilli or bolognese.

5. Don't drink much alcohol

To reduce your risk of cancer, you should limit the amount of alcohol you drink. The WCRF recommends, ideally, not drinking alcohol at all but if you must drink then limiting your consumption to no more than two units a day for men and one unit for women. One unit is half a pint of beer or a 125ml glass of 8 per cent ABV wine (see page 55).

According to Cancer Research UK, alcohol can increase the risk of seven types of cancer, including breast, liver, mouth, oesophagus and bowel cancers because it can damage DNA. Carcinogens are formed when the body breaks down alcohol. The WCRF estimates that one in five breast cancer cases could be prevented by not drinking alcohol. A 2008 study from the Breast Institute and St George's hospital, London, suggests that the increase in breast cancer observed over the last ten years is due to a corresponding rise in women's drinking. Drinking even small amounts of alcohol can increase the risk of breast cancer because high alcohol levels increase levels of oestrogen.

A review of the evidence in 2012 concluded that having one drink a day (around 1.5 units) could increase the risk of breast cancer by 5 per cent. Several studies have found that each additional unit of alcohol drunk a day increases the risk of breast cancer by 7–12 per cent. All types of alcoholic drinks, including wine, beer and spirits, can increase cancer risk. The risk is linked to the actual alcohol in the drink and increases with the amount you imbibe.

6. Cut salt

Consuming too much salt may increase your risk of stomach cancer. Studies have shown that high salt intakes can damage the lining of the stomach, which increases the chances of cancer. Limit your salt intake to 6g daily by cutting down on processed foods, especially bacon, ham, sausages, sauces, ready meals and crisps (see page 131).

7. Make time for daily exercise

It is estimated that one in nine cases of bowel and breast cancer could be prevented by being more active. Regular exercise reduces levels of hormones that cancers need to grow, such as oestrogen and insulin growth factor. The WCRF report recommends at least 30 minutes of exercise a day but the more you do and the harder you work, the greater the protection.

Try to build activity, such as walking or cycling, into your daily routine and reduce the amount of time you spend doing sedentary activities such as watching television or being on the computer. If you sit at desk all day at work, you should aim to spend at least two hours – and preferably four – a day on your feet, either standing or doing some light activity, according to new guidelines from Public Health England. This will help reduce your cancer risk. People who sit all day have a 13 per cent increased risk of cancer as well as a greater risk of heart disease and type 2 diabetes.

SIX EASY WAYS TO WALK MORE:

✓ walk short distances instead of taking the car

✓ take the stairs instead of taking the lift and walk up and down escalators

✓ set an alarm every half an hour to remind you to stand up and walk around. Spending long periods sitting down is unhealthy no matter how active you are the rest of the time

- ✓ buy a pedometer and increase the number of steps you walk each day. Aim for 10,000 steps a day, whether it's to and from work, the shops or just a stroll around the block

- ✓ when watching TV, get up and walk around during the advert breaks, and hide the remote so you have to get up to change channels

- ✓ stand or walk when you're talking on the phone – you'll burn twice as many calories as sitting

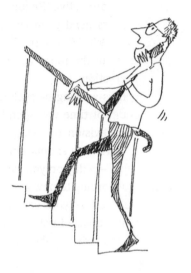

GET YOUR DAILY SUNSHINE

Getting a daily 15-minute dose of sunshine (from April to October) will ensure you get enough vitamin D, which may help protect you from bowel, breast, prostate and ovarian cancer. Most of the vitamin D in the body is created during skin exposure to UV light, but can also be obtained from oily fish and egg yolk (see page 45). Several studies have linked low blood levels of vitamin D with an increased risk of developing breast, ovarian and bowel cancer. A 2005 review of 63 studies by researchers at the University of California concluded that vitamin D could reduce the risk by as much as 50 per cent.

Protecting your skin from UV rays – even on cloudy days – is essential, not only to avoid painful sunburn but also to cut your risk of skin cancer. So it is important to wear sunscreen. Confused by the labels on sunscreens? A Royal Pharmaceutical Society report in 2015 found that most people didn't know what to look for. Buy products with both SPF and star rating or those that protect against both UVAs and UVBs. The Sun Protection Factor indicates the level of protection against UVB rays, while the star rating details protection against UVAs (which cause skin-ageing and wrinkles). Both UVB and UVA rays from the sun can cause skin cancer.

As our ability to make vitamin D from sunlight decreases with age and the National Institute for Health and Clinical Excellence (NICE) recommends supplements containing 10 micrograms (mcg) (400 IU) vitamin D each day for those over 65.

LIFESTYLE AND CANCER

According to a 2008 study from the University of California, a low fat vegan diet combined with yoga and exercise can help fight prostate cancer. Researchers found that combining a diet low in fat and rich in fruit and vegetables with regular moderate exercise seems to switch on genes that fight disease, while effectively turning off others that can promote cancer. Although this study looked at prostate cancer, the researchers believe that these findings could also be of relevance to a range of other cancers, such as breast cancer.

Osteoporosis

Osteoporosis means just what its name suggests – porous bones (or a thinning of the bones). Our bones are made up of protein (collagen) as well as calcium and other minerals. Together, these form the structure of the bone – a thick outer shell, surrounding a honeycomb-like inner core. Osteoporosis occurs when the outer shell becomes thinned. Unfortunately, our bones get thinner naturally as we become older – in fact, by the age of 75, up to half of women will have the condition. The thinning of our bones causes them to become fragile and, as a result, they break more easily. Although there's no cure, the right diet and exercise programme can help reduce your risk of fracture and slow its progress, even for people in their seventies already.

Why are women more likely to develop osteoporosis?

Women are especially prone to the disease due to a loss of oestrogen after the menopause, which speeds up bone loss, making osteoporosis more likely. In women the risk is increased if they have an early menopause, have their ovaries removed before the menopause, or miss periods for six months or more as a result of excessive exercising or dieting. For men, low levels of testosterone increase the risk.

How do I know if I have osteoporosis?

There may be no warning before a minor bump or fall causes a bone fracture, which may result in pain, disability and loss of independence. Osteoporosis may cause you to 'shrink' as you get older. It causes the characteristic 'dowager's hump'. Broken arms or wrists from minor falls can occur from osteoporosis and may give an early warning of further fractures to come. Screening tests – usually involving a bone density scan – exist, although you may have to pay for them privately. This painless test involves a low dose of X-rays (less than a normal X-ray) usually across your spine, wrist or hip. The specialist will then tell you whether you have osteoporosis, or are at risk, and will suggest treatments.

YOU MIGHT HAVE A HIGHER RISK OF OSTEOPOROSIS IF YOU:

✓ have a family history of osteoporosis, easy fractures or dowager's hump

✓ have had early menopause or hysterectomy

✓ have infrequent periods (especially linked to anorexia or excessive exercise)

✓ use corticosteroids (used to treat conditions such as asthma and eczema)

✓ are underweight (having a BMI below 18.5)

✓ take little regular physical activity

✓ drink a lot of alcohol

✓ smoke

✓ have low testosterone levels (in men)

How can diet prevent osteoporosis?
Get enough calcium

Calcium-rich foods include milk, cheese, yogurt, tinned sardines (and other tinned fish with edible bones), dark green leafy vegetables, almonds, sesame seeds, tofu and dried figs. The recommended intake is 700 milligrams a day, which you can get from three servings of dairy products (see table below). However, if you don't eat dairy products or struggle to consume enough calcium-rich foods, consider taking calcium supplements. Experts recommend taking calcium (around 400mg) and vitamin D (around 2.5mcg) supplements together. Be warned: taking more than the recommended daily dose of calcium on a regular basis could lead to heart problems and kidney stones, and interfere with the absorption of other minerals such as iron and magnesium.

TEN FOODS CONTAINING 200MG CALCIUM PER PORTION:

- ✓ 1 glass milk or milkshake
- ✓ 1 slice Cheddar cheese
- ✓ 1 small pot yogurt
- ✓ 10 sprigs broccoli
- ✓ 3 oranges
- ✓ 2 tablespoons sesame seeds
- ✓ 1½ tins sardines
- ✓ 50 almonds
- ✓ 4 dried figs
- ✓ 1 slice tofu

Boost vitamin D

Vitamin D works hand in hand with calcium and helps your body absorb it. You can get enough vitamin D from sunlight by spending 15 minutes in the sun each day between April and October (see page 44). The main food sources of the vitamin are oily fish, eggs and liver. The recommended intake is 5 micrograms (mcg) (200IU) daily but NICE recommends supplements containing 10mcg (400IU) vitamin D each day for those over 65.

Eat plenty of fruit and vegetables

Research at the MRC Human Nutrition Research in Cambridge in 2006 found that people who had the highest intakes of fruit and vegetables had a higher bone density. This may be due to the vitamin C or potassium content or other fruit-specific antioxidants, or a reduction in the production of acidity in the body with diets rich in fruit and vegetables.

Avoid fizzy drinks

Drinking cola and other fizzy drinks can lower your bone density and increase your risk of osteoporosis, according to a 2008 study involving in 2500 women. Fizzy drinks contain high levels of phosphoric acid, which leaches calcium from the bones. Researchers at Tuft's University recommend drinking no more than two of these drinks per week.

Will calcium supplements stop me getting fractures?

A 2013 review of studies concluded that there is little evidence that calcium supplements prevent fractures in pre-menopausal women or those without osteoporosis. However, for people who have been diagnosed with osteoporosis and have suffered fall fractures, doctors usually recommend supplements providing around 1000mg a day along with 20mcg (800IU) vitamin D supplements to prevent further fractures.

BUILD YOUR BONES

Your bones will be stronger if you are physically active. Weight-bearing exercises, such as walking or jogging, or playing tennis, done three to four times a week, are best for preventing osteoporosis – bones get stronger when muscles push and tug against bones during exercise. Include some strengthening and balance exercises too. They may help you avoid falls, which could cause broken bones.

Summary of Eat Yourself Well

- Many health conditions, including obesity, high blood cholesterol and high blood pressure, as well as major diseases such as heart disease, stroke, type 2 diabetes, some cancers

and osteoporosis are preventable through changing your diet
and lifestyle.

- The most important ways of cutting your risk of disease
  include maintaining your weight within a healthy range,
  taking regular exercise, not smoking and sticking to safe
  alcohol limits.
- Ways to lower your blood cholesterol level include replacing
  some of the saturated fat in your diet with unsaturated fat;
  and upping your consumption of oats, beans, lentils, nuts,
  fruit and vegetables.
- You can lower your blood pressure by switching to a
  Mediterranean diet – plenty of fruit, vegetables, fish, nuts,
  seeds, whole grains, beans, lentils and olive oil – as well
  cutting salt and losing weight if you are overweight.
- You can cut your risk of developing type 2 diabetes – or
  manage the condition if you've already been diagnosed
  - by keeping to a healthy weight, losing weight if you are
  overweight, eating plenty of fibre-rich foods (to help control
  blood sugar levels), and keeping added sugars (especially
  sugary drinks) to a minimum.
- The main diet-related ways to cut heart disease risk include
  maintaining a healthy weight and avoiding carrying excess
  weight or a paunch around your middle, swapping some of
  the saturated fat in your diet for unsaturated fats, eating a
  Mediterranean diet with plenty of fruit and vegetables, and
  sticking to healthy alcohol limits.
- You can reduce your cancer risk by changing what you eat,
  being more active and maintaining a healthy weight. In
  addition, the WCRF recommends avoiding high calorie foods
  and sugary drinks, basing your diet on plant foods, limiting
  red meat and avoiding processed meat, not drinking much
  alcohol, and cutting salt.
- Although there's no cure, the right diet and exercise
  programme can help reduce your risk of osteoporosis and
  fractures, and slow its progress. Dietary measures include
  getting enough calcium and vitamin D, eating plenty of fruit
  and vegetables and avoiding fizzy drinks.

5
RECIPES

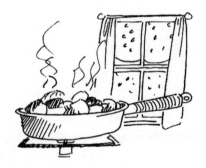

The recipes in this chapter will show you how easy it is to make delicious home-cooked food that is healthy and follows the principles of the Mediterranean diet described in Chapter 2 even if you're a novice in the kitchen. Hopefully, by now you will have a better idea about what constitutes a healthy diet and how to eat well. The traditional Mediterranean diet can be used as a blueprint for your day-to-day eating. The rules are simple. Keep sugar, salt and processed foods to a minimum. Fill up with fresh vegetables and salad, and use olive oil and butter instead of vegetable oil and margarine. Aim to fill about half your plate with fresh vegetables – always choose a rainbow of colours to get a wide range of nutrients. An easy way is to have a leafy green vegetable (like broccoli or cabbage), plus something red, orange or yellow (carrots, tomatoes, butternut squash) at the least. Your protein portion (meat, fish, chicken, eggs, beans, lentils, nuts or tofu) will then take up about a quarter of the plate and your potatoes, pasta or rice the other quarter. Choose wholegrain varieties whenever you can.

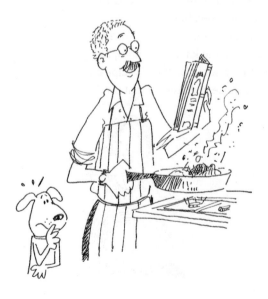

Add in a couple of pieces of fruit each day, ideally berries plus something else that's in season and you'll easily manage your seven servings of fruit and vegetables a day (page 71). Even if you're not vegetarian, try to have at least one or two vegetarian meals in a week – eating less meat and more pulses will benefit your health in so many ways.

You don't need elaborate cooking skills for these recipes nor do you need fancy kitchen equipment. If you've never followed a recipe before, you'll find it's actually quite easy, because the instructions will take you through step-by-step. All the recipes serve two, but amend the quantities accordingly if you are cooking for a different number of people. Check that you have all the necessary ingredients, then make a list of anything that you need to buy. All the ingredients in these recipes are widely available from supermarkets. Don't worry if you don't have all of them to hand. Sometimes you can create a good meal without including every single ingredient listed or by substituting, say, a different vegetable for the one listed in the ingredients.

Before you start cooking, clear the decks in the kitchen to give yourself room to work. The ingredients in the recipes are listed in order of use, so it's not necessary to weigh and prepare everything in one go before you start. You can prepare the onions, for example, for the first step and while they're cooking for 5 minutes you can prepare the next group of vegetables or trim and chop the meat. Here's a quick guide to some basic techniques before you start. No doubt some of you are whizzes in the kitchen, but hopefully a few new cooks can be encouraged to try some of these recipes, and the instructions below are written for those just starting out on their culinary journey.

Essential Kitchen Skills

How to... peel an onion

Cut the top and hairy root off the onion but leave a little of the root base so the onion doesn't fall apart. Cut the onion in half then peel off and discard the papery brown skins. Place the onion halves cut-side down on the chopping board. Make lengthwise cuts into the onion from root end to stem end. Make just a few cuts for thick slices or roughly chopped, more cuts for thin slices or finely chopped. Next, make cross-wise cuts, holding the onion firmly with your fingers.

How to... prepare a pepper

Stand the pepper on a chopping board so that the green stem is on the top. Cut the pepper in half vertically then lay the halves down. Cut out the white core and green stem with a small knife then trim away the rest of the white membrane. Rinse away the tiny white seeds under cold running water. Cut the flesh into strips or squares.

How to... peel vegetables and fruit

A swivel-bladed vegetable peeler is the easiest way to peel most vegetables and fruit. Hold the vegetable or fruit firmly in one hand or press against a chopping board. Run the peeler along the length of the vegetable or fruit, moving the blade away from you or towards you – whichever feels most comfortable. Continue until all the peel has been removed then rinse under cold running water.

How to... dice vegetables

Cut vegetables into strips. Keeping those strips together, cut across them at right angles to make small squares.

Kitchen Clean-up

Clear your cupboards, fridge and freezer of the foods you know aren't that good for you, and instead, stock up on healthy and tasty options. Here's a list of items to purge from your kitchen – and, following that, our favourite must-haves to stock up on. Donate unopened foods to a local food bank, or use up what you have on hand and then replace it with our suggestions.

Get rid of these

Throw away high-calorie, nutrient-poor foods including:

- crisps
- chocolates and sweets
- snacks (like tortilla chips and crackers)
- biscuits
- sugary breakfast cereals
- pastries and pies
- cakes
- white bread
- dips
- creamy salad dressing and sauces
- cream
- sausages and burgers
- bacon, pancetta and lardons
- canned meats
- squash, fizzy drinks and juice drinks

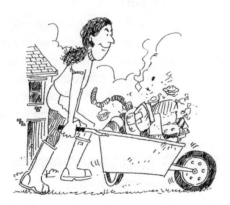

Stock up on these

Stock up on healthy and tasty options that you and your family will enjoy. Must-haves for a healthy fridge include:

- seasonal fresh fruit and vegetables
- lower fat cheeses like feta, goat's cheese, mozzarella, ricotta or small amounts of strong cheese like Parmesan for a flavour lift
- houmous

- milk and plain yogurt
- eggs
- fresh fish and small amounts of chicken, turkey and other lean meat

Fill your store cupboard with these

Food cupboard staples include:

- tinned fish such as tuna, salmon and sardines (in oil or water)
- tinned beans such as red kidney beans, chickpeas, borlotti beans, butter beans and black beans
- oats
- wholegrains such as wholewheat pasta, wholegrain rice and noodles, quinoa, barley and bulgur wheat
- dried fruit such as raisins, sultanas and apricots
- wholewheat bread, wraps, rolls, pittas and tortillas
- olives (tinned or packets fine)
- tinned tomatoes, tomato puree and passata (sieved tomatoes – widely available in supermarkets)
- nuts such as cashews, almonds, pistachios, Brazils and walnuts – unsalted
- seeds – sunflower, pumpkin, sesame
- mustard – wholegrain, Dijon, etc.
- honey and/or maple syrup to add a sweet boost to porridge
- vinegar – balsamic, sherry, red wine, white wine, etc.)
- olive oils – extra virgin, olive and light olive oil (or rapeseed oil)
- herbs and spices – rosemary, coriander, cumin, oregano, bay leaves, black pepper, basil, thyme and mint

For the freezer

Must-haves for your freezer include:

- boneless, skinless chicken breasts and fish fillets – easy everyday dinner solutions when paired with a quick salad
- bags of frozen fruits (e.g. raspberries, mixed berries) and vegetables (e.g. spinach, peas)
- portions of homemade, low-fat soups and casseroles

BREAKFASTS

It's no secret that breakfast is the most important meal of the day. In fact, research shows that typically breakfast eaters are slimmer than those who forgo food in the morning. The right breakfast foods can help you concentrate, boost your energy and help keep you feeling full until lunchtime.

Remember: all the recipes included here serve two, so amend the quantities accordingly if you are cooking for a different number of people.

Berry Porridge

Oats are packed with soluble fibre and will keep you feeling full all morning

Porridge is a comforting and healthy way to start the day. You can use other fruit instead of berries if you prefer – banana slices and chopped apple work well – and add a handful of almonds or pecans for an extra protein boost.

75g (3oz) porridge oats

400ml (14fl oz) milk (any type)

Handful of raisins, chopped dried figs or chopped dried apricots

Handful of fresh or frozen berries (defrosted)

Drizzle of honey or maple syrup (optional)

Plain yogurt (optional)

1 Put the oats into a large pan with the milk and dried fruit and heat gently, stirring until the porridge thickens and the oats are cooked, about 4–5 minutes.

2 Spoon into bowls, top with the berries, a drizzle of honey or maple syrup, and serve with extra milk or a dollop of yogurt.

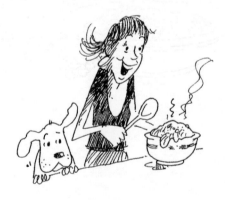

Cinnamon Porridge with Banana and Nuts

A scrumptious and healthy way to kick-start your day

If you thought porridge was boring, think again. Here's an easy and nutritious way to jazz up a bowl of oats. Add a few chopped dates or a handful of sultanas for an extra energy boost.

75g (3oz) porridge oats

400ml (14fl oz) milk

½ tsp cinnamon

1 banana, sliced

Couple of tablespoons of chopped nuts (e.g. almonds, walnuts or pecans)

1　Mix the oats, milk and half the sliced banana in a saucepan. Bring to the boil and cook for 4–5 minutes, stirring frequently.

2　Stir in the cinnamon. Serve topped with the nuts and remaining banana.

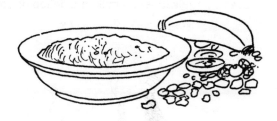

Energy-Boosting Muesli

Gives you lots of energy and keeps you going until lunchtime

This versatile muesli can easily be adapted to include your favourite fruit, seeds or nuts. There is a choice of almonds, sunflower and pumpkin seeds here, but you can add whatever varieties you fancy.

75g (3oz) porridge oats (or a muesli base)

300ml (½ pint) milk

1 tbsp sunflower seeds

1 tbsp pumpkin seeds

25g (1oz) toasted flaked almonds

Handful of fresh fruit, e.g. strawberries, raspberries or blueberries

1 Place the oats in a bowl and pour the milk over them. Leave them in the fridge to soak for at least 2 hours, preferably overnight.

2 Stir in the seeds and almonds. Serve in individual bowls, topped with the fresh fruit.

HOW TO TOAST NUTS

On their own, nuts make a delicious and healthy snack. But toasting the nuts really brings out their 'nutty' flavour. To toast nuts in the oven, spread them in an even layer on a baking tray and place in the oven at 180°C (160°C fan, gas mark 4) for 10–15 minutes. Check them often and stir halfway through the cooking time to make sure all the nuts are toasting evenly. Alternatively, toast in a frying pan over a medium-high heat, stirring frequently until they are golden brown and smell amazing. Warning: it's easy to burn them, so keep your eye on them while they're cooking. Toast a batch, store in an airtight container (or even a re-sealable freezer bag) and use as needed – they will keep for up to a month.

Bircher Muesli

Long lasting energy and packed with fibre

This is the perfect breakfast to prepare ahead of time. Make it in individual bowls and you've got breakfast ready to go, or make up a big batch and it will keep happily in the fridge for a couple of days. You can substitute the almonds for any other nuts or seeds.

75g (3oz) porridge oats

150ml (5fl oz) milk

1 tbsp sultanas

1 tbsp flaked almonds

1 tbsp honey

1 apple, grated

2 tbsp natural yogurt

1 In a large bowl, mix together the oats, milk, sultanas and seeds. Cover and leave in the fridge overnight.

2 Stir in the honey and grated apple, and serve with the yogurt.

Overnight Oats

Fruity, filling and fuss-free

Overnight Oats is an amazingly healthy breakfast made the night before and eaten straight from the fridge. Swap the berries for any other fruit you prefer – apples, melon and peach are delicious alternatives.

75g (3oz) porridge oats

400g (14oz) low fat natural or plain Greek yogurt

1 tbsp maple syrup or honey

Mixture of blueberries, strawberries and raspberries

A few walnuts (optional)

1 In a bowl mix together the oats, yogurt, maple syrup or honey and fruit. Cover and put in the fridge overnight so the oats absorb all the yogurt.

2 To serve: divide between two bowls and top with fruit and walnuts, if you like.

Blueberry and Almond Yogurt

High in protein and calcium

This is my favourite summer breakfast. It's different every time, depending what fruit there is to hand. Swap the blueberries for raspberries, strawberries or blackberries.

250g (9oz) 0% fat Greek yogurt

Tablespoon of sultanas

Handful of blueberries

Tablespoon of flaked almonds

Runny honey or maple syrup

1 Divide the yogurt, blueberries and sultanas between two bowls and mix together.

2 Scatter over the almonds and drizzle with a little honey or maple syrup. Serve immediately.

Eggs for Breakfast

Eggs pack a protein punch

Eggs are highly nutritious and are naturally rich in B vitamins, vitamin D and iron. They're inexpensive and simple to cook, especially if you know how. Just follow this step-by-step guide. Serve with wholemeal toast or a toasted bagel. Or smoked salmon, chopped avocado and some cherry tomatoes for a Sunday treat.

Again – many of you will be dab hands in the kitchen – but here's a handy recap for anyone wondering about failsafe techniques to make the perfect eggy breakfast.

Perfect Scrambled Eggs

1 Allow two eggs per person. Beat the eggs in a bowl with a fork and season with a little salt and freshly ground black pepper.

2 Melt a knob of butter in a small heavy-based pan over a low heat. Pour in the eggs and stir, using a wooden spoon to break up the lumps as they form.

3 As the eggs start to set, scrape the bottom of the pan to prevent the eggs overcooking. Scrambled eggs may be well cooked and quite firm, or soft and quite runny; this is a matter of taste. They will continue to cook even when taken off the heat, so remove them from the pan when they are still a little softer than you want to serve them.

Perfect Poached Eggs

1 Heat about 9cm (3½ in) of lightly salted water in a shallow frying pan to a bare simmer. Crack an egg into a cup and then slip it into the water.

2 Cook for 3–4 minutes until the white is just set. Remove the egg with a slotted spoon and drain on kitchen paper.

Perfect Boiled Eggs

1 Bring a small pan of water to the boil. Once the water is boiling, add the egg(s). For a soft-boiled egg, cook for 6 minutes; for a salad egg, cook for 8 minutes; and for a hard-boiled egg, cook for 10 minutes.

2 Remove the egg(s) from the water with a slotted spoon and serve.

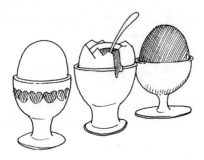

The Perfect Omelette

1 To make an omelette for one person, heat a heavy-based frying pan or omelette pan. Using a fork, beat 2 eggs and season.

2 Add a teaspoon of oil or a knob of butter to the pan, then pour in the eggs and stir a few times with a fork.

3 As the omelette begins to set at the sides, lift it up and allow the uncooked egg to run into the gap.

4 When the omelette is nearly set and the underneath is brown, loosen the edges and give the pan a shake.

5 Add a filling (such as grated cheese or sliced tomatoes), if you like, and fold the omelette in half. Slide the omelette on to a plate and serve.

MAIN COURSES

Are you fed up with meat and two veg, or just looking for a bit of healthy inspiration for main meals? Then look no further. These recipes will show you just how easy it is to turn simple ingredients into delicious and nutritious dishes. The emphasis is on lots of fresh produce, along with fish, poultry, pulses and olive oil, all of which are key features of the Mediterranean diet.

Remember: all the recipes included here serve two, so amend the quantities accordingly if you are cooking for a different number of people.

Chicken and Vegetable Pasta

Packed with vitamins and iron

This easy-to-make, tasty dish is a great source of protein, as well as fibre, iron and lots of vitamins. Feel free to use different vegetables according to what's in season. Try broad beans, asparagus and garden peas in the spring, when they're plentiful and cheap.

1 tbsp olive oil

1 onion, diced

2 skinless chicken breast fillets, cut into strips

1 garlic clove, chopped/crushed

1 courgette, sliced

1 red or yellow pepper, sliced

400g (14oz) tinned chopped tomatoes

½ tsp dried basil or mixed herbs

200g (7oz) baby spinach leaves

125g (4oz) wholewheat pasta shapes

25g (1oz) Parmesan

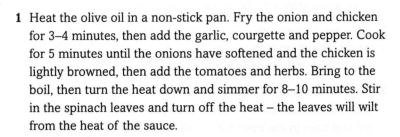

1 Heat the olive oil in a non-stick pan. Fry the onion and chicken for 3–4 minutes, then add the garlic, courgette and pepper. Cook for 5 minutes until the onions have softened and the chicken is lightly browned, then add the tomatoes and herbs. Bring to the boil, then turn the heat down and simmer for 8–10 minutes. Stir in the spinach leaves and turn off the heat – the leaves will wilt from the heat of the sauce.

2 Meanwhile, cook the pasta in boiling water according to the packet instructions, drain and return to the empty pan. Add the chicken mixture and stir to combine. Serve and scatter over the Parmesan. Serve with a rocket, spinach and watercress salad drizzled with olive oil for an extra vitamin boost.

Salmon with Roasted Mediterranean Vegetables

Rich in omega-3s

A delicious dish, easy to prepare, with very little washing up. Roasting the vegetables intensifies the flavours of this dish.

½ aubergine, cut into 1cm (½ in) cubes

1 red onion, cut into wedges

1 red pepper, chopped

1 courgette, roughly chopped

2 tomatoes, cut into quarters

2 garlic cloves, finely chopped/crushed

About 10 pitted black olives

1 tbsp olive oil

2 salmon fillets, skinned

Lemon juice

Handful of fresh basil, roughly torn

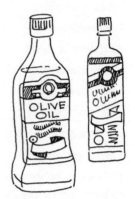

1 Preheat the oven to 200°C (180°C fan, gas mark 6).

2 Place the prepared vegetables, garlic, tomatoes and olives in a large roasting tin with the garlic. Drizzle over the olive oil and toss lightly so that the vegetables are well coated.

3 Place the salmon on top of the vegetables. Drizzle the salmon with a little extra olive oil and lemon juice. Cover the dish with foil and bake in the oven for 25–30 minutes until the salmon is cooked through and the vegetables are tender. Scatter over the basil just before serving. Serve with crusty wholemeal bread and a leafy salad.

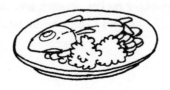

Grilled Sardines with Ratatouille

Heart-healthy dish

Ratatouille captures the very essence of Mediterranean cuisine. The tasty combination of peppers and tomatoes is brimming with vitamins A and C. When they're plentiful and cheap, use fresh tomatoes instead of tinned.

1 tbsp olive oil

1 red onion, chopped

½ red pepper, sliced

½ yellow pepper, sliced

2 garlic cloves, crushed

1 courgette, sliced

½ aubergine, cut into 2cm (¾ in) cubes

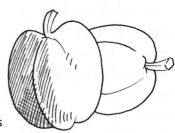

400g (14oz) tinned tomatoes

Salt and freshly ground black pepper

2 tbsp chopped fresh basil leaves or chopped fresh parsley

450g (1lb) sardines (about 8), cleaned and gutted (ask your fishmonger to do this)

Olive oil and lemon juice to drizzle

1 Heat the olive oil in a non-stick pan. Add the chopped onion and peppers and cook gently for 5 minutes. Add the garlic, courgette, aubergine and tomatoes. Stir then cover and cook over a low heat for 20–25 minutes until all the vegetables are tender. Season with a pinch of salt and some freshly ground pepper, and stir in the fresh herbs.

2 Season the sardines and cook under a hot grill for 3–4 minutes on each side or until cooked in the centre. Drizzle the sardines with a little oil and lemon juice. Serve with the ratatouille.

Chicken Tagine

Packed with protein

This warming and nutritious dish is perfect on a chilly day. It's a fantastic way of adding pulses to your meals. You could try using butter beans or cannellini beans instead of the chickpeas.

1 tbsp olive oil

4 skinless boneless chicken thighs (if you buy yours with skins on, remove before cooking)

1 small onion, finely chopped

½ tsp ground coriander

½ tsp ground cinnamon

½ tsp paprika

1 carrot, sliced

500ml (18fl oz) chicken stock, hot

½ tin i.e. 200g (7oz) tinned tomatoes

½ tin i.e. 200g (7oz) tinned chickpeas, drained and rinsed

50g (2oz) baby spinach

40g (1½ oz) dried ready-to-eat apricots, roughly chopped

25g (1oz) flaked almonds, toasted

Handful of fresh coriander, roughly chopped

1 Heat the oil in a large pan and fry the chicken on both sides until lightly coloured. Add the onion and fry gently for a further 2 minutes until softened. Add the ground coriander, cinnamon, paprika and carrots and stir well. Add the stock, tomatoes, chickpeas, spinach, apricots and plenty of seasoning.

2 Bring the mixture to the boil, then turn down the heat and simmer for 30 minutes or until the chicken is tender.

3 Stir in the almonds and coriander. Serve with couscous or brown rice.

Baked Sardines with Tomatoes and Chickpeas

The creamy 'nutty' texture of the chickpeas goes perfectly with the fish

If you can, get your sardines from a fishmonger who'll be able to debone them for you. If you buy them pre-packed, they come de-headed but you'll need to remove the backbone. To do this, use a small knife to cut a long slit underneath each fish. Lay the opened-out fish on a board, skin-side up and press gently all along the spine. Turn it over and lift the backbone away from the flesh with the side bones attached. Get rid of any fine bones with some tweezers or by gently scraping the flesh with a knife. Fold the fish back together.

1 tbsp extra virgin olive oil plus extra for drizzling

1 small onion, chopped

1 garlic clove, crushed

400g (14oz) tinned chopped tomatoes

400g (14oz) tinned chickpeas, drained and rinsed

Handful of flat-leaf parsley, roughly chopped

4 sardines, head and central bone removed

Zest ½ lemon

1 Preheat oven to 220°C (200°C fan, gas mark 7). Heat the olive oil in a large pan and fry the onion for 5 minutes. Add the garlic and fry for 1 minute more, then stir in the tomatoes and chickpeas.

2 Bring the mixture to the boil and simmer for 10 minutes. Stir in half of the parsley and season to taste.

3 Tip the sauce into a large ovenproof dish, then arrange the sardines in a layer over the sauce. Drizzle with a little oil.

4 Cook in the oven for 12–15 minutes until the sardines are cooked through. Scatter over the lemon zest and remaining parsley. Serve with crusty bread and a leafy green salad.

Easy Chicken Paella

Super simple and packed with protein

This all-in-one dish has endless variations. Use this recipe as a base for whatever fresh produce catches your eye in the shops – tomatoes, runner beans or mushrooms work well. Or make a vegetarian version by substituting the chicken and seafood for a tin of red kidney beans.

1 tbsp olive oil

½ onion, chopped

1 garlic clove, crushed

1 tsp smoked paprika and 1 tsp dried thyme

150g (5oz) paella or Arborio/risotto rice (this is plumper than American or basmati rice)

150g (5oz) chicken fillets, cut into bite-sized pieces

1 red pepper, deseeded and sliced

125g (4oz) green beans

500ml (17fl oz) chicken stock, hot

200g (7oz) frozen seafood mix (normally mussels, scallops, squid, prawns), defrosted in the fridge

50g (2oz) frozen peas

Juice of ½ lemon and handful fresh flat-leaf parsley, roughly chopped

1 Heat the oil in a large frying pan and fry the onion for 5 minutes. Add the garlic, paprika, thyme, rice, chicken, peppers and green beans and cook for a few minutes to lightly brown the chicken.

2 Add the stock and bring to the boil. Season and simmer for 30 minutes, stirring regularly until the rice is almost tender and most of the liquid has been absorbed.

3. Stir in the seafood, peas, lemon juice and parsley. Heat through thoroughly and serve.

Mediterranean Fish Stew

Easy to make and full of goodies

This is a delicious and wholesome recipe that's packed with protein, fibre, vitamins and minerals. It's a great way of adding beans to your diet – you can use chickpeas or other types of tinned beans in place of the cannellini beans, if you wish.

1 tbsp olive oil

½ onion, sliced

1 garlic clove, chopped/sliced

¼ red chilli, finely chopped

200g (7oz) butternut squash, diced

400g (14oz) tinned tomatoes

100ml (3½ fl oz) dry white wine

150ml (5fl oz) fish stock, hot

250g (9oz) skinless halibut or sea bass fillets, cut into large chunks

200g (7oz) frozen peeled king prawns (thawed)

200g (7oz) tinned cannellini beans, rinsed and drained

Handful flat-leaf parsley, chopped

1 Heat the oil in a frying pan. Add the onion and cook over a gentle heat for 5 minutes until softened. Add the garlic, chilli and butternut squash and cook for a further 3–4 minutes. Add the tomatoes and wine and cook for 10 minutes more.

2 Add the fish stock and heat until gently simmering. Stir in the halibut, prawns and chickpeas and cook for 5 minutes until the fish is opaque and cooked through and the prawns are defrosted and cooked. Then stir in the parsley. Serve with crusty wholemeal bread.

Fish with Spicy Chickpeas

Protein-rich and full of fibre

This is a great way of livening up plain grilled fish. Here it is accompanied by a tasty side dish of chickpeas and vegetables.

2 chunky white fish fillets, such as Alaskan pollock or Pacific cod

1 tbsp lemon juice

2 tbsp olive oil

1 onion, sliced

1 red pepper, sliced

100g (3½ oz) spinach

½ red or green chilli (red will be slightly hotter, especially smaller varieties), finely chopped, or a pinch of dried chilli flakes

400g (14oz) tinned chickpeas, drained and rinsed

Handful of fresh coriander, chopped

1 Brush the fish with 1 tablespoon of the olive oil and the lemon juice and cook under a medium grill for 3–5 minutes until the fish is opaque and flakes easily when pushed with a knife.

2 Heat the rest of the oil and cook the onion and pepper over a moderate heat for about 10 minutes until softened. Add the spinach and cook for a minute until wilted. Stir in the chilli. Tip in the chickpeas, heat through and season with salt and freshly ground pepper. Serve the chickpeas with the fish. Scatter over the coriander. Serve with couscous or brown rice.

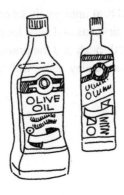

Fish Minestrone

A great source of protein and vitamins

Minestrone is a wonderful way of combining tomatoes and seasonal vegetables. Here we've added fish to boost the protein content and make it a more substantial main meal. You can use fresh or frozen vegetables.

1 onion, chopped

1 tbsp olive oil

1 garlic clove, crushed

400g (14oz) tinned chopped tomatoes

1 tbsp tomato purée

500ml (18fl oz) vegetable or fish stock, hot

50g (2oz) spaghetti, broken into short lengths

200g (7oz) vegetables (e.g. celery, leeks, carrots, green beans), chopped

150g (5oz) fish, such as haddock, cut into bite-sized pieces

1 tbsp pesto

1 Heat the oil in a large pan, add the onion and garlic and cook for about 5 minutes until softened.

2 Add the tinned tomatoes, tomato purée, stock, spaghetti and some seasoning and bring to the boil. Turn down the heat and simmer for 5–6 minutes. Add the vegetables and fish to the pan and continue cooking for another 5 minutes. Check the seasoning and serve drizzled with pesto or extra olive oil. Serve with a crusty wholemeal roll.

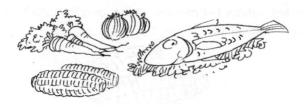

Prawn and Vegetable Stir-Fry

A tasty dish, ready in 10 minutes

Apart from being super-quick to make, this highly nutritious stir-fry provides plenty of protein as well as fibre and vitamins A and C. Cashew nuts add extra iron and monounsaturated fats.

1 tbsp olive oil

1 small onion, sliced

1 garlic clove, chopped

2.5cm (1in) piece fresh root ginger, finely chopped

1 carrot, cut into batons

½ red pepper, thinly sliced

50g (2oz) baby corn

100ml (3½ fl oz) vegetable stock, hot

50g (2oz) cabbage, shredded

100g (3½ oz) frozen cooked king prawns (thawed)

2 tbsp soy sauce

300g (10oz) straight-to-wok egg noodles

25g (1oz) cashew nuts

1 Heat the oil in a wok or large frying pan until hot. Add the onion and fry for 2 minutes. Add the garlic, ginger, carrots, pepper and baby corn. Cook for a further minute, then pour over the stock and simmer for 3 minutes until the vegetables are nearly cooked. Add the spinach and cook for 1 or 2 minutes until just wilted.

2 Stir in the prawns, soy sauce and noodles. Heat through until piping hot – about 1–2 minutes. Scatter over the cashew nuts and serve immediately.

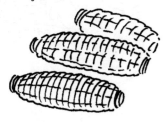

Baked Fish with Roasted Vegetables

Great source of antioxidants

White fish is rich in protein, B vitamins and minerals and in this recipe it's made even healthier by the addition of fresh tomato sauce (a great source of the antioxidant lycopene) and fresh vegetables. Substitute cubed butternut squash or aubergine for any of the vegetables suggested here.

2 white fish fillets

Half a 350g (12oz) tub fresh pasta sauce

1 yellow pepper, cut into thick strips

1 courgette, cut into chunks

4 tomatoes, quartered

1 clove garlic, crushed

1 tbsp olive oil

Handful fresh basil, roughly torn

1 Preheat the oven to 200°C (180°C fan, gas mark 6).

2 Roll up each piece of fish and secure with a cocktail stick, then place in a shallow baking dish. Pour the pasta sauce around the fish. Mix the peppers, courgettes, tomatoes and garlic in a bowl with the oil and half the basil.

3 Arrange the vegetables around the fish and cook in the oven for 20–25 minutes, or until the vegetables are tender and the fish is just cooked. It should be opaque and start to flake when tested with a fork. Remove the sticks. Serve sprinkled with the remaining basil. Serve with boiled new potatoes.

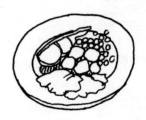

One-Pan Spanish Fish Stew

Nutritious and simple to make

This all-in-one dish combines fish, vegetables and potatoes, and so provides a near-perfect balance of protein, carbohydrate, vitamins and minerals. There are countless variations of this stew – you can use cod, haddock or monkfish or add extra prawns if they take your fancy.

1 tbsp olive oil

1 small red onion, finely sliced

1 red pepper, deseeded and cut into chunks

1 garlic clove, crushed

225g (8oz) potatoes, cut into 2cm (¾ in) chunks

200g (7oz) tinned chopped tomatoes

1 tbsp tomato puree

300ml (½ pint) fish stock, hot

225g (8oz) white fish fillets, cut into chunks

100g (3½ oz) baby spinach

Handful of fresh coriander, roughly chopped

1 Heat the oil in a pan over a medium heat. Add the onion and fry for 5 minutes. Add the red pepper, garlic, and potatoes and fry for another minute. Add the tomatoes, tomato puree and stock, season and cover the pan. Bring to the boil, then reduce the heat and simmer, partially covered, for 15 minutes or until the potatoes are just tender.

2 Add the fish, simmer for 5 minutes until it's cooked. Add the spinach and stir for 1–2 minutes until wilted. Scatter over the coriander and serve.

Sardines on Toast

Simple but rich in iron

Tinned sardines are particularly rich in iron and calcium and make a nourishing speedy lunch or supper. They're also packed with omega-3s.

2 thick slices wholemeal bread

1 garlic clove

1 large tomato, sliced

120g (4oz) tinned sardines in olive oil, drained

A little lemon juice

Handful of rocket

1 Preheat the grill. Toast the bread. Cut the garlic clove in half and rub the cut side over the surface of one side of the toast.

2 Divide the tomato slices and the sardines among the toast slices, squeeze the lemon juice over them, then put back under the grill for 2–3 minutes to heat through. Scatter the rocket over the sardines. Serve immediately, with a leafy green salad for extra vitamins and fibre.

VEGETARIAN OPTIONS

You don't need to be a vegetarian to enjoy meals without meat. In fact, it's a good idea to have at least one meal a week without it as more and more studies point to the health benefits of a plant-based diet. The traditional Mediterranean diet features only small amounts of meat but is plentiful in plant-based foods, such as beans, lentils, chickpeas, vegetables and grains. Try adding some of these recipes to your weekly repertoire.

Remember: all the recipes included here serve two, so amend the quantities accordingly if you are cooking for a different number of people.

Tofu and Red Pepper Stir-Fry

Packed with calcium and vitamins

Tofu is an excellent source of protein and calcium and can be incorporated into lots of different recipes in place of meat. Plain tofu is quite bland, so we recommend using a ready-bought marinated tofu (available in supermarkets) in this recipe for its richer flavour.

1 tbsp olive oil or rapeseed oil

1 onion, sliced

1 garlic clove, crushed

1 teaspoon fresh ginger, grated

1 red pepper, chopped

1 courgette, sliced

50g (2oz) cabbage, sliced

1 tbsp tamari (Japanese soy sauce)

125ml (4fl oz) water

200g (7oz) marinated tofu, cut into 1cm (½ in) cubes

25g (1oz) cashew nuts

1 Heat the oil in a wok until it is hot, add the onion, garlic and ginger and stir-fry on a medium to high heat for 2 minutes.

2 Add the pepper, courgette and cabbage and stir-fry for another 2 minutes. Add the tamari and water, cook for another 2 minutes then add the tofu. Leave to cook for 2 minutes. Remove from the heat and then stir in the cashew nuts. Serve with brown rice or rice noodles.

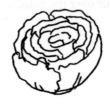

Couscous, Chickpea and Goat's Cheese Salad

Fantastic fibre boost

Chickpeas are so versatile and brilliant to add to so many dishes, including salads. Did you know they are one of the earliest cultivated crops in the Mediterranean region? Try this chickpea-infused dish for a protein- and fibre-filled meal.

125g (4oz) couscous

200g (7oz) tinned chickpeas, drained and rinsed

2 tomatoes, cut into wedges

25g (1oz) pine nuts

2 spring onions, finely sliced

50g (2oz) bag mixed salad leaves

100g (3½ oz) goat's cheese, crumbled

For the dressing:

2 tbsp extra virgin olive oil

1 tbsp balsamic vinegar

1 garlic clove, crushed

1 tsp lemon juice

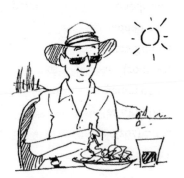

1 Put the couscous into a jug, taking note the volume, and pour into a bowl. Add the same volume of boiling water. Cover and leave for 5 minutes until the water is absorbed. Drain it and then transfer the couscous to a large bowl and stir in the remaining non-dressing ingredients.

2 To make the dressing, put the ingredients in a small screw top jar and shake well. Pour over the salad and toss to combine. Serve.

Chickpea and Butternut Squash Risotto

A great source of vitamin A and fibre

When the winter nights are chilly, this is the perfect feel-good dish. The combination of rice, butternut squash and chickpeas is warming and delicious, and the spinach and red pepper provide an extra vitamin boost.

1 tbsp olive oil

1 onion, finely chopped

1 garlic clove, crushed

½ butternut squash, roughly chopped

1 large red pepper, deseeded and roughly chopped

150g (5oz) Arborio (risotto) rice

1 litre (2 pints) vegetable stock, hot

200g (7oz) tinned chickpeas, drained and rinsed

1 sprig thyme and 3 sage leaves, chopped

Large handful rocket leaves

25g (1oz) grated Parmesan

1 Put the stock in a saucepan on a medium heat and bring it up to a simmer.

2 Meanwhile, heat the oil in a large pan over medium heat. Fry the onion for about 5 minutes or until soft. Add the garlic, butternut squash and red pepper and fry for a further 3 minutes. Stir in the rice and fry for another minute, then pour in the stock one ladle at a time. Continue adding and stirring in the stock.

3 Simmer for approximately 30 minutes until the stock is absorbed and the rice is creamy and tender (add a little water and cook for a few more minutes if the rice is a little too firm for your liking).

4 Stir the chickpeas, thyme and sage and check the seasoning. Fold through the rocket and scatter over with the Parmesan. Serve hot.

Pasta with Courgettes and Feta

Good source of fibre and protein

This simple pasta dish captures the flavours of the Mediterranean. Feta is a traditional Greek cheese made from goat's or sheep's milk and has a lower fat content than most hard cheeses. This dish is a good way of using courgettes when they're in season, but you can use other vegetables such as tomatoes, green beans or broccoli, if you prefer.

125g (4oz) wholewheat pasta shapes

2 courgettes, trimmed

1 tbsp olive oil

1 garlic clove, crushed

¼–½ tsp dried chilli flakes, to taste

Finely grated zest of ½ lemon

Handful basil, roughly chopped

50g (2oz) feta, crumbled

1 Bring a large pan of water to the boil and cook the pasta according to the packet instructions, about 10 minutes.

2 A few minutes before the pasta is due to be ready, coarsely grate the courgettes. Heat the oil in a large deep frying pan and fry the garlic and chilli for 10 seconds (watch that the garlic doesn't burn). Add the courgettes, lemon and plenty of seasoning and fry, stirring frequently, for 1 minute.

3 Drain the pasta well and add to the courgette pan together with the basil and most of the feta. Mix together and check the seasoning. Drizzle over a little more olive oil, garnish with the remaining crumbled feta and serve.

Greek Salad Wraps

Super-speedy snacks

These wraps are a great alternative to a sandwich and are just as easy to make. They're filled with a refreshing combination of fresh vegetables and feta cheese. Great for a speedy lunch.

2 tomatoes, roughly chopped

½ red onion, finely sliced

¼ cucumber, roughly chopped

6 black olives, pitted and chopped

50g (2oz) feta cheese, crumbled

2 tortilla wraps

2 tbsp houmous

1 In a large bowl, toss together the tomatoes, onion, cucumber, olives and feta to make a salad.

2 Heat the tortillas. Warm in a frying pan for 15 seconds, turning once during heating. You don't need to add any oil to the pan. Alternatively, heat in the microwave (Cat B 650W), for 10–12 seconds.

3 Spread the houmous on the tortilla. Make a row of salad down the centre. Fold in the sides to seal in the fillings and roll up tightly. Cut in half and serve immediately.

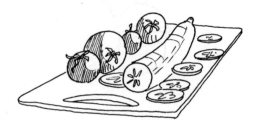

Warm Halloumi Salad

Packed with protein, fibre and iron

Halloumi is traditionally made from sheep's milk in Cyprus.
It's a firm salty cheese with a robust – almost meaty – texture
and contains less fat than most hard cheeses. When it's grilled,
barbecued or fried it becomes beautifully crispy and savoury on the
outside.

A little extra virgin olive oil

125g (4oz) halloumi

100g (3½ oz) bag mixed salad leaves

400g (14oz) tinned mixed beans, drained and rinsed

150g (5oz) cherry tomatoes, halved

Zest and juice ½ lemon

1 tsp Dijon mustard

1 Heat a griddle or frying pan over a high heat. Cut the halloumi
   into 5mm (¼ in) thick slices and brush both sides with olive oil.
   Fry for 1–1½ minutes each side until golden.

2 Put the salad leaves, beans, and tomatoes into a large serving
   bowl and toss together. Whisk together the remaining oil, zest
   and juice and the mustard. Drizzle over the salad and serve
   topped with the halloumi.

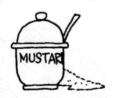

Mediterranean Pasta with Roasted Vegetables and Walnuts

Full of vitamin C and heart-healthy omega-3s

This simple combination of roasted Mediterranean vegetables, pasta and walnuts is tasty as well as a brilliant way of getting loads of vitamins. Walnuts are one of the few vegetarian sources of omega-3s, as well as a good source of protein and fibre.

½ aubergine, cut into cubes

1 onion, cut into wedges

1 red pepper, deseeded and cut into chunks

250g (9oz) small tomatoes, halved

1 clove garlic, chopped

1 mild chilli, deseeded and chopped

1 tbsp olive oil

Salt and freshly ground black pepper

250g (9oz) fresh penne pasta

50g (2oz) walnuts, chopped

Handful fresh basil leaves

1 Preheat the oven to 200°C (180°C fan, gas mark 6). Place the prepared vegetables in a roasting tin with the garlic and chilli. Toss gently in the olive oil, season and roast in the preheated oven for 20 minutes, stirring occasionally to stop the vegetables from sticking.

2 Meanwhile, cook the pasta according to the packet instructions, about 3–4 minutes. Drain the pasta and return it to the pan, mix in the roasted vegetables and walnuts. Scatter over the basil and serve in bowls with a crisp green salad.

Goat's Cheese and Beetroot Salad

Colourful, tasty and a brilliant source of vitamins and minerals

Beetroot is packed with powerful antioxidants, and has been shown to help lower blood pressure. This recipe is one of the tastiest ways of adding this super-vegetable to your diet. Add extra chopped nuts for a protein and fibre boost.

2 oranges

225g (8oz) cooked beetroot, quartered

1 tbsp fresh chives, chopped

100g (3½ oz) bag watercress, spinach and rocket leaves

100g (3½ oz) goat's cheese

For the dressing:

1 tbsp olive oil

1 tsp white wine vinegar

1 Peel and segment the oranges. In a serving bowl, mix together the beetroot, chives, watercress and orange. Crumble the goat's cheese and add to the bowl.

2 Shake the ingredients of the dressing together in a small screw-topped jar and season to taste. Toss through the dressing and serve with wholemeal crusty bread.

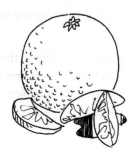

Lentil and Vegetable Dahl with Cashew Nuts

Fantastic fibre booster

Lentils make a great wholesome meal – they are nutritional powerhouses, packed with protein, fibre and iron. As an alternative you can add diced butternut squash or sweet potatoes in place of the carrots and courgettes or stir in a handful of spinach for extra iron and vitamin C.

1 onion, chopped

1 tbsp olive oil or rapeseed oil

1 garlic clove, crushed

½ tsp ground cumin, 1 tsp ground coriander, ½ tsp turmeric

75g (3oz) red lentils

400ml (14fl oz) vegetable stock

1 carrot, diced

1 small courgette, sliced

50g (2oz) frozen peas

25g (1oz) cashew nuts, toasted

A little lemon juice

Small handful of fresh coriander, finely chopped

1 Heat the oil in a heavy-based pan and sauté the onions for 5 minutes. Add the garlic and spices and continue cooking for another minute, stirring continuously.

2 Add the lentils, stock, carrots and courgettes. Bring to the boil. Cover and simmer for about 20 minutes, adding the peas 5 minutes before the end of the cooking time.

3 Stir in the cashew nuts then season with the lemon juice and salt. Finally, stir in the fresh coriander and serve.

Easy Vegetable Soup

Super-healthy and easy to adapt

Add your favourite vegetables to this simple soup – leeks, peas and butternut squash work well. If you prefer smooth soups, then simply purée with a hand blender.

1 onion, chopped

1 tbsp olive oil

2 celery sticks

2 carrots, peeled and chopped

1 potato, peeled and chopped

1 vegetable stock cube

500ml (18fl oz) boiling water

1 Heat the oil in a large saucepan over a low to medium heat and add the chopped onion, stirring occasionally. Roughly chop the celery sticks into 2cm (¾ in) pieces and add to the onion pan.

2 Add the carrots and potatoes to the saucepan and continue to cook, stirring occasionally, for another 5 minutes. Add the boiling water and crumble in the stock cube. Stir, bring to the boil then turn down again and leave the soup to simmer gently for 15 minutes.

3 Check the seasoning. Ladle into bowl or mugs. Top with cheese if you like, and serve with slices of wholemeal bread.

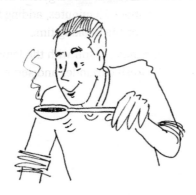

Lentil Chilli

Comfort food made from store cupboard ingredients

This easy recipe made from tinned pulses and tomatoes is full of protein, fibre, iron and B vitamins. Make it even healthier by frying diced carrots or red pepper with the onion.

1 tbsp olive oil

1 small onion, chopped

½ teaspoon each ground cumin, coriander and chilli powder

400g (14oz) chopped tomatoes

½ vegetable stock cube, crumbled

400g (14oz) lentils, drained and rinsed

400g (14oz) red kidney beans, drained and rinsed

Small handful of fresh coriander, chopped

Salt and freshly ground black pepper

1 Heat the oil in a large pan and fry the onion for 5 minutes or until soft. Add the ground spices and cook for a further minute. Stir in the tomatoes, stock cube and lentils and simmer for 10 minutes or until thickened.

2 Add the kidney beans and heat through. Stir in the coriander and check the seasoning. Serve with a simple green salad (such as rocket or watercress) and flatbreads or cooked brown rice.

DESSERTS

It's nice to round off your meal with a dessert, and it's also a delicious way of getting a serving or two of fruit. These fruit-based recipes are full of vitamins, minerals and fibre so they really will do your body good. What's more, they contain minimal or no added sugar, so you can enjoy them without guilt!

Remember: all the recipes included here serve two, so amend the quantities accordingly if you are cooking for a different number of people.

Roasted Peaches and Plums with Yogurt

Rich in antioxidants

Peaches are rich in vitamin C and beta-carotene, both of which boost your immunity and promote healthy skin, while plums are packed with antioxidant nutrients that help protect your cells from damage. This low fat dessert is perfect for summer entertaining when the fruits are plentiful and cheap.

2 ripe peaches

2 ripe plums

1 tbsp runny honey plus extra for drizzling

4 tbsp 0% fat plain Greek yogurt

1 Preheat the oven to 200°C (180°C fan, gas mark 6). Halve and stone the peaches and plums and arrange, cut sides up, in a shallow dish large enough to hold them all in one layer.

2 Pour the honey over the fruit. Roast in the oven for 25–30 minutes, basting halfway through the cooking time, until the fruit is tender.

3 Leave to cool for 10 minutes then divide between serving plates. Place a spoonful of yogurt into the cavity of each fruit and drizzle with a little extra honey if you wish.

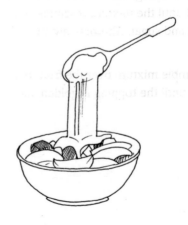

Oaty Apple Crumble

Fantastic fibre boost

This scrumptious crumble contains less sugar than the traditional version and uses oats in place of some of the flour, making it a particularly tasty way of getting extra fibre in your diet. Apples also provide lots of soluble fibre – the kind that's good for lowering cholesterol – along with vitamin C and antioxidants.

225g (8oz) cooking apples, peeled and sliced

2 tbsp runny honey

½ tsp cinnamon

2 tbsp water

For the topping:

50g (2 oz) plain flour

40g (1½ oz) olive oil spread

25g (1oz) oats

25g (1oz) brown sugar

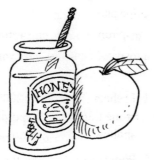

1 Preheat the oven to 190°C (170°C fan, gas mark 5). Place the apples, honey and cinnamon in a deep baking dish. Combine well and pour the water over the mixture.

2 For the crumble topping, put the flour in a bowl and rub in the olive oil spread until the mixture resembles coarse breadcrumbs. Mix in the oats and sugar. Alternatively, mix in a food mixer or processor.

3 Scatter the crumble mixture over the fruit. Bake in the oven for 20–25 minutes until the topping is golden and the fruit is tender.

Poached Plums with Ginger and Yogurt

Nutritious and delicious

Plums contain health-promoting compounds called phenols that help reduce inflammation, protect cells from damage and may reduce the risk of colon cancer. Here, plums are poached with just enough honey to counteract the fruit's sharpness and also intensify their flavour.

125ml (4fl oz) water

1 tbsp runny honey

225g (8oz) purple plums

2.5cm (1in) piece root ginger, chopped

Plain yogurt to serve

1 Place the water and honey in a saucepan and bring slowly to the boil, stirring occasionally until the honey has dissolved.

2 Halve the plums and remove the stones. Add to the honey liquor with the chopped ginger. Simmer gently for 10 minutes until the plums are tender.

3 Cover and chill in the fridge until required. Serve the plums and their liquor with a helping of natural yogurt.

Baked Apples with Dried Fruit and Nuts

Fibre-rich and full of antioxidants

This is one of the simplest yet most nutritious ways to cook apples. Here, they are filled with nuts and dried fruits, both fantastic sources of vitamins, antioxidants and fibre, and just a little honey to balance out the tartness of the cooking apples.

2 Bramley cooking apples

50g (2oz) mixture of dried fruit (e.g. raisins, sultanas, apricots, figs or dates)

2 tsp runny honey

25g (1oz) pecans or walnuts, chopped

1 Preheat the oven to 190°C (170°C fan, gas mark 5). Remove the core from the apples. Using a sharp knife, lightly score the skin around the middle, just enough to pierce the skin.

2 In a small bowl, combine the dried fruit, honey and pecans. Fill the cavities of the apples with the sticky mixture, then place them in a baking dish. They should fit snugly side-by-side. Add 2 tablespoons of water, cover loosely with foil then bake for 45–60 minutes. Serve warm with natural yogurt.

Easy Banana and Vanilla Ice Cream

No added sugar

Bananas are naturally sweet so the make the perfect base for this creamy, frozen, light dessert, which contains no extra sugar, just a hint of vanilla and a little fromage frais, to give it a smoother texture.

2 ripe bananas

1 tbsp fromage frais (or milk)

½ tsp vanilla extract

1 Slice the bananas. Transfer them to a small plastic container. Cover and place it in the freezer for at least an hour or until frozen. Alternatively, you can just pop the bananas in a plastic freezer bag and freeze overnight.

2 When you are ready to serve the dessert, place the frozen banana slices in a food processor (cut the frozen whole bananas into 1cm (½ in) chunks) with the fromage frais (or milk) and vanilla extract and blend for about one minute until smooth and creamy. You can enjoy this dessert straight away, but it will also freeze well for a day or two.

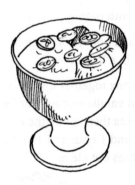

Healthy Banana Bread

Low in sugar and high in fibre

Using really ripe bananas adds natural sweetness to this delicious bread, and adding a little honey instead of sugar means it is lower in sugar than most breads and cakes. The wholewheat flour and walnuts both add extra fibre and iron to this tasty dessert.

Makes 10 slices

3 ripe bananas

3 tbsp honey

125g (4oz) self-raising flour

150g (5oz) wholemeal flour

1 tsp cinnamon

1 tsp baking powder

3 eggs

150ml (5fl oz) natural yogurt

50ml (2fl oz) light olive or rapeseed oil

1 tsp vanilla extract

50g (2oz) chopped walnuts

1 Heat the oven to 170°C (150°C fan, gas mark 3). Line a 900g- (2lb)-loaf tin with baking parchment.

2 Mash the bananas and honey together. Mix the flours, cinnamon and baking powder in a large bowl.

3 In a separate bowl, mix together the banana and honey mixture, eggs, yogurt, oil and vanilla extract. Stir into the dry ingredients along with the walnuts then spoon the batter into the tin. Bake for between 1 hour and 1 hour and 15 minutes or until an inserted skewer comes out clean.

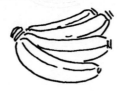

Summer Fruit Compote with Yogurt

Seasonal dessert bursting with taste, colour and vitamins

It's difficult to think of a more delicious way of getting a load of vitamins, antioxidants and fibre. Berries are rich in vitamin C as well as polyphenols that help lower blood pressure and fight inflammation. You can use fresh or frozen fruit for this recipe.

4 ripe plums, halved and stoned

Zest and juice of 1 orange

225g (8oz) mixture of strawberries, blueberries and raspberries

1 tbsp honey

Greek yogurt to serve

1 Place the plums in a small pan with the orange zest and juice and 2 tablespoons of water. Bring to the boil and simmer for 4 minutes until slightly softened. Stir in the berries and continue cooking for another minute.

2 Remove from the heat and allow to cool to room temperature. Serve with the Greek yogurt.

SMOOTHIES

Smoothies are a fantastic way of getting at least one or two servings of your daily fruit and vegetables. They contain all the vitamins, minerals, antioxidants and fibre of the whole fruit, with nothing else added and nothing taken away. Home-made smoothies are far healthier than shop-bought versions, which may contain added sugars or concentrated juice. Smoothies make a nutritious breakfast or an in-between-meal snack but, if you have a poor appetite, they are also a great way of getting lots of nutrients without making you feel to full.

Remember: all the recipes included here serve two, so amend the quantities accordingly if you are cooking for a different number of people.

Vitamin Booster Smoothie

Packed with beta-carotene and vitamin C

Cupful of crushed ice

½ mango, stone removed, peeled and diced

125ml (4fl oz) carrot juice

125g (4oz) strawberries

½ red pepper

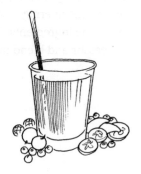

Place the ingredients in a smoothie maker, blender or food processor and blend until smooth and frothy. Serve immediately.

Healthy Heart Smoothie

Good source of antioxidants

300ml (½ pint) beetroot juice

1 apple peeled, quartered and cored

50g (2oz) blueberries

1 tbsp grated ginger

Place the ingredients in a smoothie maker, blender or food processor and blend until smooth. Serve immediately.

Strawberry Banana Smoothie

Full of vitamin C

250ml (9fl oz) orange juice

125g (4 oz) strawberries

2 bananas, frozen and sliced

First, slice the bananas. Transfer them to a small plastic container. Cover and place in the freezer for at least an hour or until frozen.

Alternatively, you can just pop the bananas in a plastic freezer bag and freeze overnight. When you are ready to make the smoothie, place the ingredients in a smoothie maker, blender or food processor and blend until smooth and thick. Serve immediately.

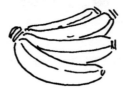

Blueberry Smoothie

Very high in antioxidants

Cupful of crushed ice
200g (7 oz) blueberries
1 small banana, peeled and cut into chunks
125ml (4fl oz) fresh orange juice

Place the ingredients in a smoothie maker, blender or food processor and blend until smooth and frothy. Serve immediately.

Cranberry Orange Smoothie

Vitamin C-rich

Cupful of crushed ice
250ml (9fl oz) cranberry juice drink
50g (2 oz) raspberries
150ml (5fl oz) orange juice

Place the ingredients in a smoothie maker, blender or food processor and blend until smooth and frothy. Serve immediately.

Strawberry and Pineapple Smoothie

Bursting with vitamin C and potassium

Cupful of crushed ice

125g (4 oz) strawberries, hulled

Half a pear, peeled, cored and roughly chopped

¼ pineapple, cored and chopped

125ml (4fl oz) fresh orange juice

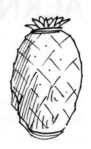

Place the ingredients in a smoothie maker, blender or food processor and blend until smooth and frothy. Serve immediately.

Breakfast Smoothie

Great vitamin and fibre booster

225g (8oz) frozen berries

225ml (8fl oz) low fat natural yogurt

3 tbsp milk

25g (1oz) porridge oats

2 tsp honey (optional)

Place the ingredients in a smoothie maker, blender or food processor and blend until smooth. Serve immediately.

ACKNOWLEDGEMENTS

The authors would like thank Charlotte Croft, Sarah Connelly and the wonderful editorial team at Bloomsbury Sport for their insights and brilliant attention to detail, without which this book wouldn't have been possible.

INDEX

Index

Index